EDITED BY
JENNY EATON DYER AND CATHLEEN FALSANI

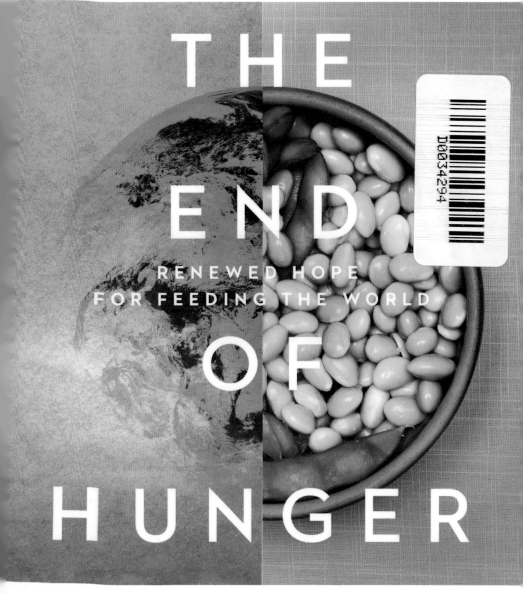

THE END OF HUNGER

RENEWED HOPE FOR FEEDING THE WORLD

WITH CONTRIBUTIONS FROM
RICK BAYLESS, TONY CAMPOLO, WILLIAM H. FRIST,
TONY P. HALL, RUDO KWARAMBA-KAYOMBO,
MIKE MCHARGUE, KIMBERLY WILLIAMS-PAISLEY AND
BRAD PAISLEY, JEFFREY D. SACHS, AND MORE

"The amazing array of voices gathered in this book will begin with good news about the progress we've made in addressing hunger since 1990. They'll share the hard news about what hunger is and what it does to human brains, bodies, and souls. Then, they'll invite you to be part of creating more good news, so you know how you can be a part of the growing global movement to end hunger—in our lifetime."

Brian D. McLaren, author, speaker, and activist

"Every generation of Christians has to ask themselves how they will respond to the global issues of their day, to the challenges taking place on our watch. *The End of Hunger* hosts a coalition of voices: global experts, activists, storytellers, and men and women for whom hunger and food insecurity have been their lived experience. Together they offer wisdom and practical insight toward a multifaceted response to global hunger. Furthermore, they issue a clarion call to use our voices, our love, and our lives to make a difference. The time and opportunity is now. *The End of Hunger* is a must-read!"

Jo Saxton, author, speaker, cohost of Lead Stories podcast

"Deeply moving and insanely motivating, *The End of Hunger* reminds us that we have more power than we ever imagined to change the world. This is the book that will spark a revolution of everyday activism that will bring about the eradication of hunger and malnutrition. Through beautiful storytelling and impressive research, the message of hope shared in these pages will surely invigorate your soul and change your perspective on what is possible."

Mandy Arioto, president and CEO of MOPS International

"A magnificent book, which couldn't come at a better time. It brings together a host of voices that explain, reveal, inform, inspire, and encourage, all in the interests of carrying out an urgent task that all people of goodwill can agree on: feeding the hungry."

James Martin, Jesuit priest, author of *Jesus: A Pilgrimage*

"Everywhere that I work in rural Africa I see the loss of life and potential as a result of malnutrition. Sadly, global hunger most often affects those most vulnerable—children and young mothers. *The End of Hunger: Renewed Hope for Feeding the World* is a clear reminder of this problem from the unique perspective of many: scientists, health care workers, advocates, those from the community of faith, and those directly affected by global hunger. The book both inspires with evidence of the progress that has been made, and challenges with a call for all of us as followers of Jesus to keep our hearts of compassion open and to continue to do what we can to heed Jesus' words, 'When I was hungry, you gave me something to eat.' "

Paul Osteen, missionary surgeon, associate pastor, Lakewood Church, Houston, TX

"Once again Cathleen Falsani and Jenny Eaton Dyer deliver a thoughtfully curated canon of truthful revelations and authentic epiphanies. Brilliantly weaving confessional mean-derings with imperative treatments of hope, the range of voices is remarkable—activists and chefs, social scientists and theologians, politicians and musicians. *The End of Hunger* is not only timely but an urgent appeal to heal the world by healing what's broken in each of us. This book offers a practical roadmap for mending these aches."

Christopher L. Heuertz, author of *The Sacred Enneagram* and founding partner of Gravity, a Center for Contemplative Activism

"This book is an important and thoughtful look at one of the most serious problems across the world. Each of the essays treats hunger with equal parts compassion, equity, justice, and ultimately hope, showing us the way forward in building a better world. Proper nutrition is a right and a key element of what people of all faiths and creeds are called to do in caring for the most vulnerable. Hunger is therefore more than a relief, development, and advocacy issue; that there are hungry and starving people is a moral issue and a religious matter. I am grateful for this resource and the challenges it poses as well as the answers it offers."

Jim Wallis, editor in chief of *Sojourners* magazine and president of Sojourners, author of *America's Original Sin*

"We must remember the Beatitudes are both spiritual and social wisdom. The call to 'hunger and thirst for righteousness' is also a call to come together and ensure everyone has food at the table. In the Franciscan tradition we remember that creation is the first Bible, and we can see there is enough to go around while many are yet hungry. *The End of Hunger* shows us the way to get there by 2030."

Richard Rohr, OFM, Center for Action and Contemplation

"'Love,' as one contributor to this book states, 'is at the root of justice.' In this collection, we're given a clear call to action—as well as simple and achievable steps that every one of us can take—to transform our love for God into hopeful and effective advocacy on behalf of vulnerable populations. After all, what did Christ tell his dear and blunder-prone friend Peter to do as a sign of his love? 'Feed my sheep.' I'm grateful for this compelling book; may it rouse each of us into action."

Jennifer Grant, author of *Maybe God Is Like That Too* and *Maybe I Can Love My Neighbor Too*

"My favorite kind of leadership is one that ignites a spark of fire deep within the belly and shows us exactly how to fan the flames of that ambition to set the world ablaze. That's exactly what this book delivers. By bringing together this collection of voices from thought leaders, advocates, and activists of every stripe, *The End of Hunger* lays out real-life stories of individuals impacted by the hunger crisis, food scarcity, and malnutrition and tells us in practical terms how we can make a global difference in this fight just by incorporating a few simple dial turns and adjustments from where we do life. Whether it's the choices we make from the aisles of our grocery store, or what we harvest from the vegetable garden growing in the back yard, or how we engage in our community and with our elected officials, or the way we feed and nourish our loved ones and have conversations with them around the dinner table, everyone can have a seat at the table in this work. I really believe that *this* is the stuff that matters, and it's what is going to change the world."

Jen Hatmaker, author of *For the Love* and *Of Mess and Moxie* and host of the For the Love podcast

"To grow, cook, eat, and share food is to participate in God's nurturing ways with the world. To consign anyone to hunger is not just to condemn them to a miserable life. It is also to deprive them of one of the most visceral and basic experiences of God's love. This is why Christians must do everything they can to understand the causes of hunger, and then eliminate them one by one. Read this book and discover how you can become a vital member in God's daily work of providing for every creaturely need."

Norman Wirzba, Gilbert T. Rowe Distinguished Professor of Theology, Duke Divinity School, author of *Food and Faith: A Theology of Eating*

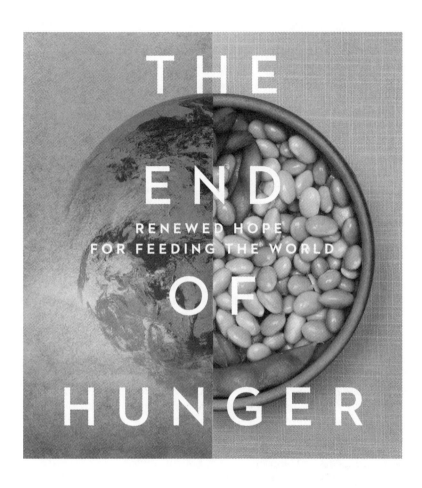

THE
END

RENEWED HOPE
FOR FEEDING THE WORLD

OF
HUNGER

EDITED BY
JENNY EATON DYER AND CATHLEEN FALSANI

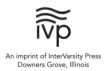

An imprint of InterVarsity Press
Downers Grove, Illinois

InterVarsity Press
P.O. Box 1400, Downers Grove, IL 60515-1426
ivpress.com
email@ivpress.com

InterVarsity Press® is the book-publishing division of InterVarsity Christian Fellowship/USA®, a movement of students and faculty active on campus at hundreds of universities, colleges, and schools of nursing in the United States of America, and a member movement of the International Fellowship of Evangelical Students. For information about local and regional activities, visit intervarsity.org.

All Scripture quotations, unless otherwise indicated, are taken from The Holy Bible, New International Version®, NIV®. Copyright © 1973, 1978, 1984, 2011 by Biblica, Inc.™ Used by permission of Zondervan. All rights reserved worldwide. www.zondervan.com. The "NIV" and "New International Version" are trademarks registered in the United States Patent and Trademark Office by Biblica, Inc.™

While any stories in this book are true, some names and identifying information may have been changed to protect the privacy of individuals.

Jeremy K. Everett, "Remember Us When You Come into Your Kingdom" essay, excerpted and adapted from the author's chapter "The Americans" in the forthcoming title I Was Hungry, *©2019 Brazos Press. Used with permission of Brazos Press, Grand Rapids.*

Cover design and image composite: David Fassett
Interior design: Jeanna Wiggins
Images: blue watercolor: © kentarcajuan / E+ / Getty Images
green beans: © Johner Images / Getty Images
planet Earth: © Vitalij Cerepok / EyeEm / Getty Images

ISBN 978-0-8308-4571-2 (print)
ISBN 978-0-8308-6569-7 (digital)

Printed in the United States of America ⊗

Library of Congress Cataloging-in-Publication Data
A catalog record for this book is available from the Library of Congress.

P 25 24 23 22 21 20 19 18 17 16 15 14 13 12 11 10 9 8 7 6 5 4 3 2 1

Y 37 36 35 34 33 32 31 30 29 28 27 26 25 24 23 22 21 20 19

FOR THE 815 MILLION PEOPLE

IN THE WORLD TODAY LIVING WITH HUNGER—

because everyone has the right

to good nutrition.

CONTENTS

INTRODUCTION

JENNY EATON DYER

S ince 1990, our generation and our nation have led the world in halving the number of people who live in extreme poverty around the world, and we did this in spite of the population growth during this time period.[1] Cutting extreme poverty in half has equated to cutting hunger in half. This is historic. This is epic. Among the many things, good and bad, for which our generation will be remembered, this is a brilliant moment for us.

Not only have we been able to tackle extreme poverty and hunger, but also—during this same time period—we have halved the number of deaths caused by HIV/AIDS, tuberculosis, and malaria, as well as maternal mortality and child deaths (under the age of five). With a united front of forces including governments, coalitions, the private sector, foundations, philanthropic organizations, and the faith community, millions of lives have been saved from extreme poverty and disease.

We are halfway to defeating extreme poverty and disease worldwide.

Through agreed-on sustainable development goals led by the United Nations, we have come together as nations to learn how best to solve some of the world's biggest challenges—including hunger. The good news is that we are succeeding. We are on course. And we know, scientifically, politically, and spiritually, what it will take to move forward to end hunger by 2030. Zero hunger is the second of seventeen goals, and we can achieve this goal by rethinking how we grow, share, and consume our food on this planet.[2]

This book is about the second half of this journey, a renewed hope for feeding the world. It is dedicated to those who live with hunger and its deleterious effects throughout their lifespan. We lift up these people and their voices to you to better understand their suffering and their hope for a better tomorrow. In doing so, we provide five vignettes of individuals who have lived with or live with the reality of starvation or malnutrition.

Our book opens with an overview of the problem of hunger. With leading experts, from those on the front lines of famine to politicians, economists, theologians, and scientists, we cover the problems of global hunger and malnutrition. Hunger is complicated, involving layers of issues from the individual to the conflicts between nations. We must take these various systemic causes seriously if we are going to truly address the roots of the problem.

Next, through a juxtaposition of stories and science, we unfold one of the latest scientific advances to overcoming the lifelong cognitive and physical consequences of malnutrition: addressing nutrition in the first one thousand days of a child's life—from the moment of conception to the child's second birthday. During this sacred period, science has shown that if the mother and the child can obtain the full spectrum of proper nutrients, which include micronutrients such as iron, protein, folate, and other vitamins and minerals, the child can avoid stunting, which can cause poor physical growth of the body and the brain. Children who experience stunting live with higher rates of chronic illness, less education, and fewer job opportunities during adulthood. Nutrition during the first one thousand days not only affects the life of the child, but it also causes a ripple effect to impact their family, community, society, and ultimately the nation.

Finally, we offer a way forward. What can we do as citizens, perhaps even as Christians, living in the United States today? How can we play a role in ending hunger? In providing nutrition during the thousand-day window for a mother and child? Our authors suggest a variety of responses from growing your own garden, to cooking at home, to fasting, to advocacy.

Advocacy is the often-overlooked Christian practice of speaking up on behalf of the poor. We ask you, our readers, to reconsider the power of advocacy by lifting your voices to let our congressional leaders know that you care deeply about how our nation provides for the world's most vulnerable populations. With less than 1 percent of our US budget, we provide the world's leading amounts of funding to tackle extreme poverty and disease. The majority of this funding for global health goes to addressing HIV/AIDS, tuberculosis, and malaria. Nutrition funding, unfortunately, receives only a fraction of this amount and has remained stagnant for decades.

We need to reconsider nutrition, its importance in the Sustainable Development Goals (SDG), its critical role in addressing global health and development, and the amount of funding we, as a nation, are willing to spend to end hunger and malnutrition worldwide.

Your voice and your will to end hunger will be a lynchpin in the coming years on whether or not our generation will be able to say we didn't only halve hunger—we ended it.

Will you join us?

PART 1

AN OVERVIEW OF THE PROBLEM OF HUNGER

HUNGER AND YOUR BRAIN

Feed the Hungry. You'll Feel Better Too.

MIKE McHARGUE

When I die, the coroner will probably write "pizza" on the death certificate as my cause of death. My devotion to food and eating doesn't end with those miraculous, savory pies we call pizza. I start to fantasize about lunch about an hour after breakfast. Dinner springs to mind by about two in the afternoon. My life is completely centered around mealtimes, and there's no recurring train of thought in my life more common than, "What am I eating next?"

If I miss a meal by more than a few hours, my usually sanguine disposition evaporates. In doing so, an acrid bed of irritability and confusion is exposed. To paraphrase Bruce Banner, "You wouldn't like me when I'm hungry."

So, it probably comes as no surprise that I've never managed to make it more than a few hours into a spiritual fast without giving up. Years ago, as I trained for a marathon, I carried food with me, so I could snack as the hours rolled by, and my feet went numb. Still, for someone who *feels* hungry all the time, I have no idea what it's really like to be *actually* hungry. None at all.

Hunger is a complex biological process, and I've only experienced its beginning stages. Those start in the stomach. A couple of hours after your last meal, your stomach begins to contract in order to sweep any remaining food into your intestines. Sometimes, this causes a rumble or two, which are called borborygmus. Once the stomach is emptied, your insulin and blood sugar levels start to drop, and the body responds by producing a hormone called ghrelin.

Ghrelin stimulates the hypothalamus in your brain. The hypothalamus is buried deep within your brain and regulates some of our most basic bodily functions, such as sleep, thirst, and sex drive. In response to the ghrelin message, the hypothalamus produces a neurotransmitter—neuropeptide Y—that you experience as appetite.

So, you eat.

I choose pizza most of the time, but you may have a healthier relationship to food than I do. The body has a couple of systems to help you feel full, involving the hormone leptin and the vagus nerve, but don't worry about that. Just know that as long as you eat every six to eight hours, your hunger cycle is quite shallow.

That's because you don't deplete your glycogen stores. You're restocking those shelves before they run dry, and you're able to keep producing glucose on demand—which is great. Your brain basically runs on glucose. Twenty-five percent of the glucose your body uses goes to your brain.

But what happens when you don't eat for longer than six to eight hours? Well, you run out of glycogen and get "hangry," or hungry-and-angry. I know all about *hangri*ness, and I'm insufferable when I reach this state.

By the time you reach this point, your body enters a metabolic state called ketosis where it starts burning fat stores instead of glucose.

When your body burns fat, it produces fatty acids, which are much larger molecules than the glucose your brain usually consumes. They're so large, in fact, that they can't cross the blood-brain barrier at all. Your brain recognizes there's no glucose available and starts to consume ketone chains instead, which are derived from the fatty acids that come from burning fat cells.

If you've heard of the keto diet, that's a fad designed to make your body think it's starving. You don't have to be starving to be in a state of ketosis: low-carb diets and intense or endurance exercise can get you there. And, ketosis does burn fat—but at a cost. Only about 75 percent of the energy your brain needs can be supplied by ketosis.

Depending on how long you sleep, and how many hours before bed time you ate, it's entirely possible to go into ketosis while you sleep. This state of ketosis can play a role in feeling foggy or less sharp than normal. Your cognitive functions are impaired while you're in a state of ketosis.

What happens when you go even longer without eating? After seventy-two hours or so, your body changes strategies. Your brain needs glucose, and your body breaks down protein into amino acids, which can then be transformed into glucose.

But if you aren't eating, where can your body get this essential protein?

From your muscle tissue and internal organs—including your heart. That's where. Then your bones start to lose density as well. If you don't eat for a week or two, you become so depleted of vitamins and minerals that your immune system starts to shut down.

When you're starving, there's a good chance that an opportunistic infection will kill you before starvation does. If an infection doesn't get you, perhaps cardiac arrest or organ failure will.

This is why I say I don't know what hunger is like. I've only ever experienced the normal appetite of someone who is well-fed. I've never had to break down muscle tissue to keep my brain going, or had my immune system start to shut down because of malnutrition.

But, one in nine people living on this planet right now is intimately familiar with hunger—*actual* hunger. They go to bed hungry most of the time.

This kind of chronic hunger is physically debilitating. Imagine you have just enough food to keep yourself in a nearly constant state of ketosis, with a brain so starved for glucose that it asks the body to perform cellular autocannibalism.

Think about the kinds of enduring hardships that are required for a person not to eat. Who would choose such a thing? It takes a natural disaster or utter economic stagnation for most of us in the developed world to miss very many meals in a row.

And yet, more than 700 million people worldwide are hungry, starving, or malnourished.

Science can describe hunger and starvation with startling clarity. But, it also can measure the amount of food required to feed the world—and, of course, we already grow enough food to feed every person living on Earth. What we're lacking is not the capacity to produce food, but the will to make sure the food we grow makes it into hungry bellies everywhere.

●   ●   ●

As a Christian, I am grieved by hunger. The Bible is absolutely packed with admonishments for those with plenty to share what they have with those who don't have enough. The poor. The hungry. The homeless. The prophet Isaiah put it like this:

> If you spend yourselves in behalf of the hungry
>   and satisfy the needs of the oppressed,
> then your light will rise in the darkness,
>   and your night will become like the noonday." (Isaiah 58:10)

In the New Testament letter that bears his name, James says our faith is dead if we refuse to meet the physical needs of others. This is from the second chapter of the Epistle of James: "Suppose a brother or a sister is without clothes and daily food. If one of you says to them, 'Go in peace; keep warm and well fed,' but does nothing about their physical needs, what good is it? In the same way, faith by itself, if it is not accompanied by action, is dead" (James 2:15-17).

Proverbs says it particularly poignantly: "The generous will themselves be blessed for they share their food with the poor" (Proverbs 22:9). If you're thrown off by the "bountiful eye," then think of the Gospel of Matthew, which says, "The eye is the lamp of the body" (Matthew 6:22). Often when Scripture speaks of our eyes, it's talking about the condition of our character, or even our souls.

We don't need biology to understand how horrific starvation is—the authors of our Holy Scriptures knew, and told us that God is pleased when we share what we have to feed others.

We have plenty of food to feed everyone. So, in a world where American Christians have incredible, even historic, wealth—how can so many people go hungry?

I can think of more than 700 million reasons.

Our brains work best when we are trying to understand or comprehend communities of around 150 people. Any time you get people together in a group that is small enough for each person to know everyone else, we humans can be remarkably altruistic. The kinds of polarizing social labels we use to divide ourselves in social conflict don't hold up in smaller groups.

We may bristle when people describe themselves as "liberal" if we see ourselves as "conservative," and we may even demean and degrade each other on Facebook or Twitter. But in person, when we can see the facial expressions and body language emerge from the object of our scorn, it tends to melt away rage and replace it with something else: empathy.

The more someone is hurt, the more we can see their pain, the more empathy we feel. If we insult someone and they look sad, or cry, we can't maintain our anger. We feel their pain. If someone is injured, we respond even more readily. And who, when faced with a person obviously starving to death, could turn them away?

Very few of us, indeed.

But when I tell you that more than 700 million people in the world are hungry, that's a scale your empathy isn't equipped to handle. Even if that bit of information prompts you to think deeply about the problem, your empathy will swell to the point where you become overwhelmed and, therefore, unable to act. Paralyzed. Imagining hundreds of millions of starving children doesn't usually motivate us. Instead, we shut down as our brains try to defend themselves through emotional defense mechanisms.

Now, if you're a person who never thinks about the hungry, it's time to do so. Make an effort to open your mind, and your heart. But, if you're a person who feels overwhelmed or even grieved by the magnitude of hunger in our world, I have great news. There's a scientifically proven solution to make you feel better: *take action*.

When you take some meaningful action to help others, including giving to charity and contacting elected officials on behalf of people in need, your brain releases several substances that neuroscientists call the "happiness trifecta": oxytocin, serotonin, and dopamine.

In today's world, that trifecta can be hard to come by. We're surrounded by a twenty-four-hour news cycle, geopolitical strife, and ever-deepening polarization. But, when we help, really and truly help, we push back the fog of anxiety, sadness, and anger, and we experience true joy.

Shifting our lives in this way has profound health benefits. When we help others, we don't just make their lives better—we feel better too. You may find that it's easier to maintain a healthy weight and that you are at a lower risk for heart attack or stroke when you take action to help others.

We are designed to help others. And we are built to give to others. Our culture may tell us that happiness comes from buying things, or taking exotic vacations, or looking beautiful and sexy. But that's a lie.

Modern science and our faith are in total agreement that true joy belongs to those who help those in need.

You can feel better. Right now.

Just turn to the Next Steps section of this book. There you'll find a list of actions—practical steps you can take to help alleviate hunger.

Pick one and do it.

And do it now. (You can thank me later.)

THE END OF HUNGER

JEFFREY D. SACHS

T he end of hunger will come when everybody on the planet enjoys an adequate basic income, has access to healthful foods, and lives in a safe environment that ensures sufficient and reliable food production.

The challenge, therefore, is to overcome poverty, malnutrition, and environmental degradation. It's a tall order, but it is feasible. More than that, in a world that is rich enough, technologically capable enough, and aware enough to take on these complex challenges, it is our moral imperative.

The world's governments have agreed to do just this—at least on paper. They have adopted seventeen Sustainable Development Goals (SDGs) that address the direct and indirect challenges to ending hunger by 2030. They include the following:

Goal 1: End poverty in all its forms everywhere.

Goal 2: End hunger, achieve food security and improved nutrition, and promote sustainable agriculture.

Goal 3: Ensure healthy lives and promote well-being for all at all ages.

Goal 4: Ensure inclusive and quality education for all and promote lifelong learning.

Goal 5: Achieve gender equality and empower all women and girls.

Goal 6: Ensure access to water and sanitation for all.

Goal 7: Ensure access to affordable, reliable, sustainable, and modern energy for all.

Goal 8: Promote inclusive and sustainable economic growth, employment, and decent work for all.

Goal 9: Build resilient infrastructure, promote sustainable industrialization, and foster innovation.

Goal 10: Reduce inequality within and among countries.

Goal 11: Make cities inclusive, safe, resilient, and sustainable.

Goal 12: Ensure sustainable consumption and production patterns.

Goal 13: Take urgent action to combat climate change and its impacts.

Goal 14: Conserve and sustainably use the oceans, seas, and marine resources.

Goal 15: Sustainably manage forests, combat desertification, halt and reverse land degradation, and halt biodiversity loss.

Goal 16: Promote just, peaceful, and inclusive societies.

Goal 17: Revitalize the global partnership for sustainable development.

These goals present a clear roadmap for the world. We share this road, all of us making our ways to the future, and it behooves us to try harder to get there together and well.

Here are the facts: about one billion of the world's 7.6 billion people live in extreme poverty, and most of the poor also are hungry. (The World Bank poverty measure suggests that 766 million people were living with extreme poverty in 2013.[1] Because there are multiple definitions of poverty that yield roughly similar numbers, one billion living with poverty is a good, rough estimate.)

For many people globally, low income means they are unable to ensure a regular and nutritious diet. Another one billion or so live above the extreme poverty line, but nonetheless are undernourished and suffer from chronic deficiencies of one or more micronutrients including iron, folates, vitamins, or healthful fatty acids. Another one billion or more are malnourished with diets overly rich in sugar, refined grains, and processed meats, resulting in obesity and metabolic diseases such as diabetes. (The overweight population globally is at 1.9 billion, and the obese population at more than 650 million.[2]) The rough estimates give us the scale of the challenges.

At the macro level, looking at the world as a whole, there is no reason why hunger and poverty could not be ended. As is well known, the world grows enough food for 7.6 billion people, yet because of vast differences in incomes, there are also vast differences in access to a healthy diet. The first cure for hunger is to ensure that everybody has an income high enough to obtain the food they need. This basic income would combine their market earnings with transfers from government as necessary to lift them above the poverty (and hunger) line.

Transferring income from the rich to the poor in order to ensure that everybody has sufficient purchasing power to feed themselves and their family would not be difficult. The world's total income each year is now on the order of $88 trillion, or roughly $11,500 per person.[3] That's certainly enough for anyone to enjoy an adequate diet, as well as adequate shelter, clothing, schooling, health care, electrification, safe water and sanitation, and other basic needs. But of course, this $11,500 average is distributed between rich countries, with incomes averaging above $50,000 per person, and countries such as those in the Sahel of Africa with incomes averaging less than $1,000 per person.

Roughly speaking, there are about one billion people in the rich countries and one billion people in the poor countries. If the rich countries transferred just 1 percent of their annual income to the poor countries, they would bolster the incomes of the poor by about $500 per person per year—enough to eradicate hunger.

The rich countries have long promised to give 0.7 percent of the national income as Official Development Assistance (ODA, meaning assistance from governments). Another 0.3 percent should come from private philanthropy, for a total of 1 percent per year from the rich countries to the poor countries. Yet the US government falls woefully short. The US ODA is only 0.18 percent of US income, or therefore 0.52 percent (=0.7–0.18) of national income less than it should be.[4] The shortfall from the US federal government alone is $100 billion per year.

Note also that there are only 2,208 billionaires in the world today.[5] Mainly in the rich countries, these billionaires have a combined net worth of $9.1 trillion. If they gave just 1 percent of their net worth, a small fraction of their annual incomes, toward the world's poorest billion people, that would amount to almost $100 per person—a major step toward ending poverty and hunger.

●　●　●

No one should argue that aid is the long-term solution to poverty. No individual person—and no country—wants to live off the largesse of others. Economic development is within reach for all countries, especially if the rich countries help the poor countries to finance the infrastructure, schooling, and health care to raise productivity. In other words, development aid is a temporary measure until the national incomes of the poor countries rise through better schooling, better health care, better infrastructure, and more home-grown businesses.

Hunger problems around the world are exacerbated dramatically by poor nutrition. America's food industry literally is killing us, and it is rapidly spreading its damage around the world. The American food industry has created a diet that is obesogenic, meaning it is a major cause of the obesity epidemic that has left *70 percent of American adults overweight (BMI > 25) and 40 percent obese (BMI > 30)*.[6] The main culprits are sugar additives in countless fast foods, sugar-based beverages, refined flour, and processed meats. This unhealthy diet is addictive, and made more so through relentless advertising that links these unhealthy foods with seemingly attractive lifestyles.[7] Another aspect of America's unhealthy diet is excessive consumption of meat, which at around 120 kilograms per year is the highest meat consumption in the world. Excessive meat consumption is linked to increased cardiovascular disease and some cancers.

Beef consumption also puts a very heavy pressure on the environment. As is well known, every kilogram of feedlot beef requires around ten to fifteen kilograms of feed grain to raise each head of cattle, a heavy burden on arable land and freshwater supplies. Moreover, increased cattle grazing is no solution, as the expansion of cattle ranching is a major cause of deforestation and land degradation. And yet, when America's nutritionists tried in 2015 to warn Americans that their heavy beef diet was contributing both to ill health and to environmental stresses, *our then Secretary of Agriculture sided with the US meat lobby and shut down the nutritionists*.[8] In America, the status quo is to choose profits relentlessly over health and environmental safety.

One part of ending hunger is ensuring that incomes everywhere are adequate to afford a healthy and nutritious diet. The second is ensuring that what we eat is healthy. The third is protecting the environment to ensure a secure and stable global food supply.

• • •

Industrial agriculture is, in many ways, its own worst enemy. The food sector has contributed massively to global warming through deforestation (which releases carbon dioxide into the atmosphere), and through the release of greenhouse gases throughout the food supply chain. It has been estimated that agriculture as a whole is responsible for about one-quarter of the total human emission of greenhouse gases (the gases that are warming the planet). The keys here are to reduce beef production and consumption, use fertilizer and water far more efficiently, and shift, in general, from grains and meat production to other proteins, including legumes, vegetables, fruits, and other parts of the diet with a much lighter environmental load.

But stopping the environmental damage of the food sector itself is only part of the solution to an environmentally secure food supply. "It is time to rethink how we grow, share and consume our food," the description of the second Sustainable Development Goal says.

> If done right, agriculture, forestry, and fisheries can provide nutritious food for all *and* generate decent incomes, while supporting people-centered rural development and protecting the environment. Right now, our soils, freshwater, oceans, forests and biodiversity are being rapidly degraded. Climate change is putting even more pressure on the resources we depend on, increasing risks associated with disasters such as droughts and floods. Many rural women and men can no longer make ends meet on their land, forcing them to migrate to cities in search of opportunities.[9]

"A profound change of the global food and agriculture system is needed if we are to nourish today's 815 million hungry and the additional 2 billion people expected by 2050," the UN Sustainable

Development Goals read. "The food and agriculture sector offer key solutions for development, and it is central for hunger and poverty eradication."[10]

We must end our reliance on fossil fuels more generally, in order to put a halt to increasingly disastrous human-induced global warming. *Temperatures are already soaring to levels not experienced during the entire period of civilization, the past 10,000 years.*[11] The results include a dramatic increase in heat waves, droughts, floods, extreme tropical cyclones, and other climate-related hazards. Food supplies in many parts of the world are under rapidly increasing levels of stress. Environmental refugees also are on the rise. Only a dramatic and rapid decarbonization of the world energy system—that is, a shift from coal, oil, and gas to wind, solar, geothermal, hydro, and other zero-carbon energy sources—can protect us from the consequences of human-induced climate change.

We can identify many other environmental threats to food security. Soils are being degraded by poor farm practices and poisoned by pesticides and other chemicals. Freshwater supplies are being used far faster than they are recharging. Nitrogen and phosphorus-based fertilizers are concentrating in coastal areas, causing eutrophication and dead zones in more than one hundred estuaries around the world. Invasive species introduced by poor agricultural practices are causing upheavals in ecosystems. Overfishing is depleting major fisheries. Trade in endangered species is driving many large animals to the brink of extinction. Large classes of animals, including pollinators such as bumblebees, are being deprived of habitat or killed via pollution and climate change, to the dire detriment of agriculture itself.

This, then, is the paradox of our age. The ability to end poverty and hunger is within reach—if we only try. Yet the ability to wreck our health and degrade our planet are just as real and immediate.

The fate of the planet should not be a guessing game, a matter of odds, or a gamble. It is a moral choice. Jesus was right to emphasize that feeding the poorest among us constitutes the ultimate moral judgment of our actions. May we choose wisely the road before us for our own lives and the life of our planet.

A THREAT TO HEALTH
ANYWHERE IS A THREAT
TO PEACE EVERYWHERE

WILLIAM H. FRIST

I n 2011, I traveled with then Second Lady of the United States Jill Biden to the DaDaab refugee camp in Kenya where hundreds of thousands of Somalis had fled, seeking to escape the worst famine the region had seen in sixty years.

The desperation, hardship, and loss suffered by these refugees was overwhelming. Many had walked for weeks, often barefoot, with few or no belongings, in search of food and medical care. Children were particularly vulnerable. On this long journey, many parents had watched helplessly as their children lost their lives to starvation.

We heard from one mother who was too weak to carry both of her children, so she was forced to make the heart-wrenching decision to leave one behind with the hope of saving the other.

It was a trip I will never forget.

In the months prior to our arrival in Kenya, the international community had begun to mobilize, and it made a difference in saving lives. But it should not take a catastrophic famine to rally our nation and the global community around the goal of ending hunger and malnutrition. Too often, the aid and support are short-lived.

It's a story we've experienced before. In the 1980s, we saw the horror of the Ethiopian famine. We watched Sir Bob Geldof raise money with LiveAid, and we listened to American musicians sing "We Are the World." And amid the seemingly countless infomercials pleading for our help and the onslaught of news coverage of the famine, we became numb. We developed what is known as "famine fatigue" and shut our eyes and ears to the issues of malnutrition and hunger.

Sadly, malnutrition still accounts for nearly half (45 percent) of all child deaths under age five.[1] Twenty-two percent of children are stunted due to poor nutrition.[2] And every four seconds, someone dies from hunger or hunger-related causes, often a child. A shocking 821 million people suffer from various forms of malnutrition and undernourishment worldwide.[3]

But there is good news. I saw this level of devastation before in 1997 when I traveled with Samaritan's Purse to treat patients in war-torn Sudan. At the time, the AIDS epidemic had taken hold of the country, and a generation of mothers, fathers, teachers, doctors, and builders had been wiped out. At its peak, the disease was killing three million people globally—that's more people than died in the entire Korean and Vietnam Wars combined—every year. It had escalated to a global public health crisis; that is, until the United States government mobilized to intervene.

Through visionary, compassionate leadership, President George W. Bush proposed, and we in Congress passed, the President's Emergency Plan for AIDS Relief (PEPFAR). This legislation provided an unprecedented 15 billion dollars to fight AIDS throughout Africa and the developing world—more than any country has ever committed to fight a single disease.

American industry also stepped up. Our remarkable scientists got to work, and together, they developed powerful, life-saving, anti-retroviral drugs. In Africa, infected teachers and workers regained health to build stronger and more secure communities. In Botswana, for instance, life expectancy jumped from thirty-nine years to sixty-seven.[4] Today, PEPFAR directly supports the antiretroviral treatments for more than 14.6 million of the 21.7 million people living with HIV.[5] They are alive today thanks to the medical innovations advanced by the United States' herculean commitment.[6]

Perhaps even more remarkably, if lesser-known, is PEPFAR's role as a powerful "currency for peace." PEPFAR-recipient nations saw the health of their people return, which facilitated a reduction in political instability and violence, improved rule of law, and increased economic output per worker. It had strategic diplomatic benefits, improving these nations' views of the United States compared to similar non-PEPFAR regional countries, and fostering new trading partners. Our investment did more than save lives; it revitalized whole nations while improving America's national security and global standing.

The passage of the landmark PEPFAR legislation in 2003 cemented our legacy of global leadership. For the past sixteen years, we have led the world in curbing pandemics of epic proportion including HIV/AIDS, tuberculosis (TB), and malaria. Very soon we may turn the corner, and these infectious diseases may be a thing of the past—if we maintain our leadership of funding for just a few more years.

And yet, with a laser focus on disease, we have overlooked a critical lynchpin of global health: hunger. We responded so boldly to the HIV/AIDS crisis because we viewed the disease as a health emergency that could take the lives of tens of millions and destroy the fabric and stability of communities, countries, and even whole regions. While malnutrition is not a complex disease like HIV/AIDS or TB, it kills more people every year than AIDS, malaria, and tuberculosis combined.[7] It deserves the same bold leadership and the commitment of resources.

Yet, the present US administration has shortsightedly recommended draconian cuts of more than 30 percent to the US foreign assistance budget. Hope Through Healing Hands (HTHH), a global health organization I founded fifteen years ago, has called on Congress to reject the White House's cuts. Together with public health advocates, faith leaders, academic researchers, nonprofit leaders, and others we stood on the front lines and advocated for the restoration of funds to the international affairs budget, including the global health account that covers issues such as vital HIV, malaria, and tuberculosis prevention and treatment, along with clean water and nutrition for vulnerable families. Through letters, phone calls, and in-person advocacy, we reminded elected officials of the critical importance of supporting the world's most vulnerable populations, particularly mothers and children.

A 2016 World Bank study found that 70 billion dollars in nutrition-specific financing worldwide is needed from 2016 to 2025.[8] An investment of this magnitude would save the lives of an estimated 3.7 million children, result in at least sixty-five million fewer stunted children, lead to 265 million fewer women suffering from anemia, and result in 105 million more children exclusively breastfed over 2015 figures. This investment in a generation of mothers and children would combat chronic disease, enhance capacity for increased education, and lead to better job opportunities in the years to come. Melinda Gates calls this investment "jumpstarting a virtuous cycle," which leads individual people, families, communities, and nations out of poverty.

Now is not the time to cut America's modest global health funding. As Martin Luther King Jr. said, "Injustice anywhere is a threat to justice everywhere." With health as the touchstone of a nation's stability, prosperity, and well-being, a threat to health anywhere is a threat to peace everywhere.

We have the data showing us the right thing to do. We have the bilateral and multilateral mechanisms ready to increase access to nutritious foods worldwide. Because policy often follows politics, we need to renew the will of the American people to remind their members of Congress and the current administration that increased funding for nutrition is the smartest and most cost-effective investment to save lives, promote peace, and enhance sustainability.

Simply put, you don't go to war with someone who has just saved the life of your child.

Global hunger is a problem on which we as a nation can turn the tide, and investments in maternal and child nutrition, in particular, will help build the foundation for subsequent generations to survive and thrive. A mother should never have to make the decision about which of her children to feed and give a chance at life.

Together, we can make a meaningful difference in the lives of millions by helping those who lack basic nutrition. Tackling this challenge will serve as a shining example of US global leadership at its best and demonstrate the unparalleled compassion of the American people.

THE BIBLE, POVERTY, JUSTICE, AND CHRISTIAN OBEDIENCE

RON SIDER

A bout fifty years ago, I had a disturbing conversation with Frank Gaebelein, a prominent evangelical Christian leader who had been a coeditor at *Christianity Today* and the headmaster of perhaps the most prominent evangelical Christian prep school in the nation.

Dr. Gaebelein, who had become actively involved in the early years of Evangelicals for Social Action as we sought to raise the issues of poverty and justice, told me that in more than half a century of attending evangelical Bible conferences, not once had he heard a sermon on justice.

Surely that isn't the experience of everyone in all parts of the Christian church now (or then), but I fear it remains true that too few pastors and church leaders in any part of the Christian community talk as much about poverty and justice as the Bible does.

There are literally hundreds and hundreds of references to it throughout Scripture.[1] So in this chapter, I want to lay out what I believe the Bible tells us about three related topics that are essential for any discussion of hunger and malnutrition:

1. God's special concern for the poor;

2. sin as both personal and social; and

3. a definition of economic justice.[2]

GOD AND THE POOR

The Bible underlines God's special concern for the poor in at least four ways: God acts in history to lift up the poor and oppressed. God identifies with the poor. God casts down rich people who oppress or neglect the poor. And people with resources who fail to share God's concern for the poor are not really God's people at all.

Accounts of the Exodus in the Old Testament repeatedly say that God acted in part to end the poverty and oppression of the Israelites (Deuteronomy 26:5-8; Exodus 6:5-7). In the New Testament, Jesus describes a central part of his mission this way:

> The Spirit of the Lord is on me,
>> because he has anointed me
>> to proclaim good news to the poor.
> He has sent me to proclaim freedom for the prisoners
>> and recovery of sight for the blind,
> to set the oppressed free. (Luke 4:18)

Second, God identifies with the poor in an astounding way. Oppressing the poor insults God (Proverbs 14:31), but "whoever is kind to the poor lends to the Lord" (Proverbs 19:17). Jesus actually taught that when we feed the hungry and clothe the naked, we minister to Jesus himself (Matthew 25:35-40).

Third, the Scriptures frequently teach the disturbing truth that God casts down the rich and powerful when they acquire their wealth through oppression, or when the rich fail to aid the poor. In the Magnificat, Mary praises God because God has "brought down rulers from their thrones . . . [and] sent the rich away empty" (Luke 1:52-53). And James warns the rich to "weep and wail" for their impending judgment (James 5:1). Why were they judged harshly? Because they were not paying their workers fairly.

Time and again, the Bible denounces those who get rich by oppressing others. The prophet Jeremiah bluntly proclaims that God would punish the rich because they had become "rich and powerful" by preying on others (Jeremiah 5:26-29; see also Jeremiah 22:13-19). In a similar way, Isaiah declares God's judgment against the rich and powerful: "It is you who have ruined my vineyard [a metaphor for the people of Israel]; the plunder from the poor is in your houses. What do you mean by crushing my people and grinding the faces of the poor?" (Isaiah 3:14-15).

Elsewhere, the Bible recounts how the rich were on the receiving end of divine punishment simply because they were wealthy and did not help the poor. According to Ezekiel, that was the reason for Sodom's destruction (Ezekiel 16:49-50).

If we become rich through oppression or are rich and refuse to use our resources to empower the poor, the God of history actually is working against us.

Fourth, perhaps the most astonishing aspect of God's special concern for the poor is this: the Bible declares many times that people who refuse to share God's concern for the poor are not really God's people at all—no matter how orthodox their creeds or how intense their religious activities may be.

Amos says God hated and despised the people's cultic activities because they were trying to worship God and oppress the poor at the same time (Amos 5:21-24). Isaiah declares that God rejected the people's fasting because "on the day of your fasting, you . . . exploit all your workers" (Isaiah 58:3).

Jesus was even more plainspoken, saying that those who do not feed the hungry and clothe the naked depart eternally from the living God (Matthew 25:41-46).

God does not love the poor more than the rich. But virtually all rich and powerful people love themselves much more than the poor.

Our human biases make it appear (to us) as if God's lack of bias is actually a bias in favor of the poor. It isn't. But make no mistake: God's lack of bias does not mean that God is neutral in historical situations of poverty and oppression. Precisely because God loves everyone equally and, therefore, demands that poverty and oppression end, God acts in history on the side of the poor and oppressed to end their poverty and oppression.

People who want to follow what the Bible teaches will seek to allow what Scripture so clearly says about God and the poor to shape how they preach, teach, and live.

PERSONAL AND SOCIAL SIN

By "personal sin," I mean things such as lying, stealing, and committing adultery. By "social sin," I refer to participation in unjust societal systems such as slavery, apartheid, institutionalized racism, and unfair economic systems.

In the past few decades, the way different preachers preached (if they talked about sin at all) illustrated a striking division. Theologically conservative preachers typically focused on personal sins, whereas more theologically liberal preachers tended to emphasize social sins.

But the Bible seems to care about both! The prophet Amos declares that the nation of Israel would go into captivity because of its sin:

For three sins of Israel,

even for four, I will not relent.

They sell the innocent for silver,

and the needy for a pair of sandals.

They trample on the heads of the poor

as on the dust of the ground

and deny justice to the oppressed.

Father and son use the same girl

and so profane my holy name. (Amos 2:6-7)

In the first section, the prophet clearly condemns economic oppression. Selling the innocent for silver and the needy for a pair of shoes refers to unjust courts where the rich bribe the judges, using the judicial system to oppress poor people. Their denial of justice to the oppressed is like stomping their heels into the ground. But the prophet then immediately adds that sexual sin is also why God will destroy the nation. Similarly, the prophet Isaiah denounces both those who seize the land from poor peasants and those who are drunkards (Isaiah 5:8-9, 11, 22-23).

The Bible is clear that laws themselves can be oppressive and unjust. The Psalmist denounces wicked rulers who "frame mischief by statute" (Psalm 94:20-23 JB). Or as the New English Bible translates the passage, they contrive evil "under cover of law." Isaiah bluntly attacks legislators who write unjust laws:

Woe to those who make unjust laws,

to those who issue oppressive decrees,

to deprive the poor of their rights

and withhold justice from the oppressed of my people. (Isaiah 10:1-2)[3]

When they think about poverty, many Christians fixate on personal causes and solutions. They may be willing to provide food baskets or disaster relief, but they are far more reluctant to examine the underlying structural causes of poverty. The great Catholic advocate of the poor, Bishop Dom Helder Camara of Brazil, famously said: "When I give food to the poor, they call me a saint. When I ask why the poor have no food, they call me a Communist."

Giving a hungry man a fish is good. Helping him learn how to fish, so he can feed himself (and others) for a lifetime, is better. And in order to fish for a lifetime, poor persons need to be able to access the ponds. The problem we face today is that many of the world's ponds are controlled by just a few extremely wealthy people who don't like to share. Structural change is required to correct the social sin of such unjust economic arrangements.[4]

A DEFINITION OF ECONOMIC JUSTICE[5]

One way the Bible helps us develop a definition of economic justice is through the discussion of land in the Old Testament. While there is no extended, systematic treatment of economic justice per se, what the Bible says about land can help us formulate a definition.

Israel was an agricultural society. And in an agricultural society, land is the basic capital—the fundamental means for creating wealth and making an adequate living. The way Israel handled the proper division of land differed sharply from surrounding societies. In Egypt, the Pharaoh and the temples owned all the land. In other Near Eastern societies, a feudal system prevailed where the king gave a few powerful people huge tracts of land that in turn were worked by poor, landless peasants.

But in Israel, the ideal was for each family to own its own land. Joshua 18:1-10 and Numbers 26:52-56 describe how, after Israel entered the land of Canaan, the land was divided so that every family received some.[6]

According to numerous biblical texts, God wanted this pattern of decentralized land ownership to continue. Leviticus 25 (one of the more radical economic texts in the Bible) decrees that every fifty years, the land reverts back to its original owners—no matter how or why they have lost their land. If practiced, this provision would have prevented the consolidation of land in the hands of a few powerful persons.

But that is exactly what happened under the kings of Israel. Again and again, the prophets denounced rich people who seized (often "legally" by bribing judges) the land of poor people. The prophet Elijah denounced King Ahab for abusing royal power by seizing Naboth's ancestral family land (1 Kings 21). Isaiah attacked rich landowners for seizing more and more of the land of smaller farmers (Isaiah 15:5-8). In fact, the prophets declared that God would punish the nations of Israel and Judah with destruction and captivity precisely because of their economic oppression and idolatry (see Micah 3:1-4, 9-12; Isaiah 1:21-26; Jeremiah 7:1-15; 12:1-7).

Strikingly, however, the prophets also imagined a future messianic time when justice once again would prevail and "everyone will sit under their own vine and under their own fig tree, and no one will make them afraid" (Micah 4:4; see also Zechariah 3:10). In that future time of justice, everyone again would possess their own land, without fearing that the rich and powerful would take it from them!

The biblical ideal is a decentralized economic ownership where neither the state nor a few wealthy persons own all the land (and therefore the society's basic capital). Instead, every family has its own land, which it can work responsibly to earn an adequate living.

This arrangement suggests a basic definition of economic justice. God wants every person and family to have access to the productive resources (that is, "capital") so that if they act responsibly they make enough to cover their needs and be dignified members of their society.[7]

Today, while there are areas where land remains the most basic capital, the most important capital in a knowledgeable society is a good education. Christians who seek to implement the biblical ideal of economic justice must work to guarantee that every person in the world has access to the physical and intellectual capital they need to earn a decent living.

To do that we must face two stubborn facts. First, our global market economies produce the luxury goods people with money want and allow the poor with no capital or money to die of starvation or disease. Second, at least two billion people live in extreme poverty with virtually no capital. They have no land, little or no access to education, and almost no money. So, if we want to implement a biblical standard of economic justice, we must work to restructure dramatically today's economic arrangements so that every person and family has access to land, loans, and school. Wise redistribution (especially via educational systems that are at least as good for the poorest members of society as they are for the wealthiest) is essential.

A FAITHFUL CHRISTIAN RESPONSE

While we have made major strides in combating extreme poverty globally, today two billion people still struggle to survive on two dollars (or less) a day.

Christians need to change. Our personal lives. Our churches. Our society.

First, we need to live more simply so that the poor may simply live. The vast majority of Americans are wealthy in comparison to the two billion poorest people on the planet. We easily could decide to spend significantly less on ourselves so that we can give more to effective programs that promote economic development for our poor neighbors around the world.

Second, our churches need to change. Every pastor and church leader must ask themselves: Am I talking and preaching about the poor as much as the Bible does? And if not, is my job security, rather than Jesus, my Lord?

Third, we all need to be involved in a small group or community where members have developed sufficient trust to help each other think about how we should spend our money in light of global poverty and the overwhelming biblical teaching about God's special concern for the poor.

Finally, we need to change the structures of our society. We need to work more vigorously and effectively to correct the weaknesses of market economies; make international trade and international corporations fairer; preserve the environment; and guarantee that foreign aid is both more extensive and more effective.[8]

Each of these tasks is complex and complicated. Invariably, Christians will reach differing conclusions about what the best, specific strategies may be. But we must start with the clear biblical teaching that faithful Christians must work tirelessly to promote economic justice. Then we must inform ourselves with the best studies, data, and expertise from leading economists and development specialists about which programs are most effective.

If we do that, over the next two decades, Christians can contribute dramatically to bringing about the end of global poverty.

A MULTIPRONGED
APPROACH

RUDO KWARAMBA-KAYOMBO

W hen I think about global hunger, I recall the many faces I've encountered during the past fifteen years of working in development and advocacy across the African continent: from Zimbabwe, to Uganda, to countries in southern Africa (Angola, Democratic Republic of the Congo, Lesotho, Malawi, Mozambique, Swaziland, South Africa, Zambia), and beyond.

ZIMBABWE

My earliest encounters with hunger were in Zimbabwe between 2001 and 2003, when a famine spread across at least five countries in southern Africa, with Malawi, Zambia, and Zimbabwe at the epicenter. An image that will never leave my mind is from an area called Matabeleland, a province in southern Zimbabwe. There, near the town of Bulawayo, I went to a food distribution site and was amazed by the number of elderly women who were queued up to receive food.

The biggest group of old ladies I had seen in my life was a graphic manifestation of the confluence of hunger, HIV/AIDS, and a missing generation. The aged were left to care for their orphaned grandchildren or the children left behind when their parents went to neighboring Botswana or South Africa to look for work.

A food distribution site remained their only hope for a meal—for themselves and the many children in their care. When we would speak with them—sometimes through an interpreter, because the local dialect was foreign even to me—they would say, "We're so thankful to God that he sent you," as if we were some kind of saviors. We were not, of course. But we were helpers and allies, sent to assist them in dealing with the effects of food scarcity resulting from crop failure, water stress, and lack of resources.

•   •   •

Hunger manifests in different ways. It can be total lack of food, but it also can be an incapacity to grow enough food, or to buy what a family needs for its ongoing sustenance. There can be hunger that is vivid and confronts us like a smack in the face. But hunger also can be less obvious—a simple lack of capability to meet one's ongoing food needs.

I'm a lawyer and a humanitarian, not a livelihood expert. But when I worked as part of an army of aid organizations that came to rescue the millions who were without food, I began to understand the effort it takes to paint the picture of the need, raise the resources to meet the need, and then set up systems to make sure that food assistance reaches the people who need it most.

In 2003, Stephen Lewis, then the United Nations' Special Envoy for HIV/AIDS in Africa, visited southern Africa to learn more about the devastating famine afflicting Zimbabwe, Lesotho, Swaziland, Malawi, and Zambia. Lewis witnessed how the HIV/AIDS epidemic caused many farmers in the region to die, so that when drought struck, communities had neither the labor force nor the water sufficient to produce food.

That famine was my first experience with the ways the humanitarian community categorizes and prioritizes those who are in need. In 2003, there were those who received food simply because they were in a particular geographical area where crops had failed. There were others who received food because their caregiver was elderly and simply didn't have the capacity to grow any food.

Then there was yet another category: those who received food aid because they were either undergoing treatment for tuberculosis or were infected with HIV/AIDS, and they needed additional nutritional support to cope with their complex medical issues.

UGANDA

In 2010, I came face to face with a totally different manifestation of hunger. This was in Uganda among the Karamojong—a pastoral people who live in the northeastern part of the country. They are cattle keepers and don't devote much attention to producing grains. They move from place to place in search of pastureland and water.

One of the unique issues of such a pastoral community is that they don't produce sufficient cereal crops. By 2010, they had been receiving food aid for more than forty years.

I was with World Vision at the time, and we were working with the Karamojong to try to boost the production of small crops. But, you see, when you introduce something like that, you're asking people to alter their way of life. It isn't in them to become farmers. And that's when hunger strikes—when their primary currency, which is their cattle, dies off because of a severe drought and the mismanagement of natural resources. During that time I learned that the Ugandan government had created a park that encroached into the pastoral lands of the Karamojong, curtailing their primary method of coping with drought: their nomadic lifestyle.

This way of life sustains them. When you restrict their movement, you might as well have taken food from their plates. Sadly, we have yet to make progress.

●　　●　　●

In the spring of 2018, I was in Ethiopia at the Tana Forum, a gathering to discuss peace and security across Africa. There we heard a new report on the nature of conflict in the Sahel, the horn of Africa, and in parts of central Africa.

The conflict there hinges on a failure by society to understand the livelihoods that support pastoral communities. The report, titled "New Fringe Pastoralism," noted that pastoral people are not new, but that they've been pushed farther onto the fringes of society by encroachment onto their land as well as by the effects of climate change.

As we are struggling to deal with the hunger issue, we keep coming up against new dynamics. First, it was HIV and AIDS and their impact. Then came climate change with its extreme weather patterns—flooding in one part of a region while there is drought in another.

And now it's pastoralism—a way of life under threat. This has caused conflict to flare up, and when it does, people are often quick to label the conflict as religious. Maybe it's Muslims against Christians, or cattle keepers against the growers of grain.

But the conflict isn't primarily sectarian or even ideological. It's a fight for scarce resources. When such tension erupts in physical conflict, any means of constructive dialogue or constructive activity really seizes, because conflict throws everything into an ungovernable community. No one has time, space, or security enough to be productive. Conflict only widens and deepens the circle of hunger.

To reach the Sustainable Development Goal of ending global hunger by 2030, we would need to use all the tools that are at our disposal. Through my work with World Vision, and now with ONE, I've learned that some of those tools involve building household resilience and giving people different strands of livelihoods. For example, if they're a crop-growing community, you introduce other ways of boosting their household economy so should there be extreme weather patterns and their crops fail, they have another way of coping. Likewise, if they're a pastoral community, we would help them find other means, or make sure no one is trying to compel them to resort to ranching their animals, or any other lifestyle they could not adjust to.

Then we need to understand what's behind their vulnerability, and address it—community by community, dealing with the unique drivers of the hunger that are unique to their people group, lifestyle, and way of life.

A multipronged approach that is contextually appropriate has the best chance of success. And in more stable communities, preventing hunger might mean coming alongside people to enhance their coping mechanisms, such as dealing with extreme weather conditions.

In some communities, combating hunger might mean helping women in small villages learn savings and loan skills so that they can grow their small businesses and not be wholly dependent on farm production. They might also learn to do some bartering and acquire the food they need that way.

SWAZILAND AND ETHIOPIA

What do we do in the year of plenty in order to prepare for the years of scarcity? We know something is coming our way. Why is it that over and over again we're caught off guard? That is the major challenge of our time.

It's mid-2016 in Swaziland. Cattle are dying. There is no water. Once again, the United Nations sends an envoy—this time human rights champion Mary Robinson, the former president of Ireland and United

Nations High Commissioner for Human Rights from 1997 to 2005. She comes to Swaziland and visits some of the sites, and we see some of the work that's being done to help communities that are under stress—water stress, food stress—to grow some vegetables to diversify their diet. All well and good.

But a few weeks later, I went back to Swaziland, and I went to a food distribution center. I was introduced to two girls who I accompanied home to see why they were in a queue for food. I learned that their mother had gone across to South Africa to look for work, leaving these two teenage girls to fend for themselves.

Oh, my goodness! We had gotten an early warning from the Famine Early Warning Systems Network.[1] We knew that southern Africa was about to be hit by another drought. Why didn't we move cattle to places that still had grazing? Why didn't nations get together and work with large-scale farmers and move cattle from one place to another? Why didn't we encourage farmers to sell on time and slaughter their cattle while they still had something to sell?

Zimbabwe alone lost at least 16,500 head of cattle during the 2016 famine.[2]

One definition of insanity is doing the same thing over and over again and expecting the result to be different. How do we stop such an insidious cycle?

Africa has the potential to feed the world, but without agriculture, it will not be able to rise to that potential.

At the 2014 African Union Summit in Equatorial Guinea, the heads of state of all fifty-five nations on the African continent agreed in the Malabo Declaration to commit at least 10 percent of their public expenditures to agriculture, in order to ensure "its efficiency and effectiveness" as part of a larger plan to end hunger in Africa by 2025.

In Addis Ababa, Ethiopia, in January 2018, I attended a presentation about how many countries are actually meeting the Malabo commitment to agricultural investment. Very, very few are. It's a failure of policymaking because the countries that are meeting the 10 percent target—and even exceeding it—are seeing their agricultural sector being transformed.

Ethiopia, for example, has put countless tracts of land under cultivation. And they're beginning to produce the food that they need so that we never have to go back to witnessing starving Ethiopian children as we did during the terrible famine of the 1980s.

The many African countries that are not meeting the Malabo goals lack the political will to do so. We continue to elect policymakers who are seated in big offices lining their own pockets. They lack empathy for the people they've been elected to serve. If they had empathy, they would invest the required amount to turn around agricultural production, health systems, and education.

Sadly, we know that "corruption kills more people than AIDS, TB, and malaria combined," as ONE cofounder Bono said during his 2016 testimony before the US Senate Appropriations Subcommittee on State, Foreign Operations, and Related Programs.

RWANDA

Those who benefit from corruption will not willingly change their ways until a demand is created by citizens. In order for there to be more open governments and more transparent systems and processes, there will have to be a coalition of the willing who begin to model what is possible.

Many things are said about President Paul Kagame's complicated legacy, and about Rwanda as a country. But I recently spent a weekend there and whatever else may be happening in that country, there is progress. It's visible, it's tangible.

Since the international community's failure in 1994 to stop the genocide in their country, the Rwandese people have been taught that they are their own saviors. They are their own security. They are their own developers. Take charge and change where you are, and the change will become what we live.

The driver who was taking me to the airport in Kigali said to me, "In this country, people have been told and told—do not wait for somebody else. It's up to us to change our destiny."

And in many ways, Rwanda has. It is being hailed for having achieved a 30 percent representation by women in its parliament. Right now, Rwanda's minister of finance is a woman; its minister of agriculture is a woman. And Rwanda produced the former director of the African Development Bank, Donald Kaberuka. Rwanda is producing people who are making a difference—and they're willingly sharing those people with continental bodies, so that the difference can begin to spread wider than just Rwanda. Political will is the key ingredient.

●　　●　　●

What then might ordinary US citizens do to help bring about change in Africa and elsewhere to bring about the end of hunger? It's important for Americans to understand that we are a globalized world—that people who are hungry, people who are on the fringes of society, need those of us who have a little bit more to give of our money and our voices.

Our money, so that those who are involved in turning that money into real help can reach those in need through food aid, medicine, or education. Our voices, in order to put our weight behind campaigns that look for both sides of the corruption. Corruption happens in Africa because somewhere in North America or in Europe or in the Middle East, someone else makes it possible for corrupt leaders to hide their money, or there are people who are willing to pay bribes to get contracts in Africa at the expense of entrepreneurs and industry that is Africa-based.

Any campaign that is worth its salt in the coming days will look at the two sides: What can African leaders do differently, and what can African citizens call their leaders to do differently? Likewise, what can leaders of the first world, the northern world, the developed world do differently, and what can citizens in the developed world call for their leaders to do differently?

It must be a global compact, because we are each other's keepers. We all share a planet, and the responsibility to manage the earth and natural resources. Environmental management still is seen largely as an expert area. But it needs to be brought into the center of our education systems. Civic responsibility, what it means to be a citizen of the world, needs to be integrated into our education system.

SOUTH AFRICA

In April 2018, I attended a memorial service for Winnie Mandela where Bishop Malusi Mpumlwana, who founded the anti-apartheid Black Consciousness Movement in South Africa, said, "An accountable government is the product of an active citizenship."

Our activity as citizens must be grounded in an understanding of what it means to be responsible citizens. The tagline for the ONE Campaign is, "None of us are equal until all of us are equal." It's all those things that we need to really think about and really own and really live. And we need to be people who will, over and over and over again, ask ourselves for more on behalf of another.

If we are to see the end of global hunger, we must change the mindset of our generation—young and old. When we talk about "all hands on deck," it should be *all* hands. All of them. Everybody.

And the world cannot wait.

ONWARD TO 2030

WILL MOORE

There is one thing that most Americans still seem to agree on: our world is increasingly on a downward spiral. Americans cite a range of issues as evidence of this spiral including economic hardship for many in the United States, the outbreak of diseases like Ebola and Zika, the horrible images of war coming out of Syria, and the threat of terrorism at home. For many who read disturbing stories like these on their news feeds every day, it feels almost like the end times. A recent survey asked Americans, "In general, do you think that people's quality of life around the world has gotten better in the last ten years, gotten worse, or hasn't really changed?" Only 7 percent said they believed the world was getting better.[1]

The problems now facing our country and our world are real and troubling. But if you actually compare human life today to human life in recent history, the truth is that by most measures, human life today is significantly better.

Incredibly, over the past twenty-five years, our world has actually cut global poverty, global hunger, and global undernutrition in half. Each and every day this year, nineteen thousand fewer children will die than on each day in 1990.[2]

In 1960, more than twenty million children under the age of five were dying every year. Today it's fewer than six million.[3] Moreover, the global population of children younger than age five has more than doubled between 1960 and today. So, we have twice as many young children on the planet today, but more than fourteen million fewer child deaths each year compared to sixty years ago. Behind each of these numbers is a child who will live to celebrate his or her fifth birthday, and who will almost certainly have greater access to education, health care, and economic opportunity than at any other time in human history.

This improvement is due in large part to global development efforts: to the expansion of markets, to the proliferation of new technologies, and to billions of dollars of investment in human health and development by philanthropists, churches, donor governments such as the United States, and increasingly by low- and middle-income country governments themselves.

The good news is that while malnutrition and hunger have in many ways been humankind's oldest story, what has happened in virtually an instant in the context of human history is startling. A true miracle has occurred right under our noses, and nobody is talking about it. Nobody is spreading the good news. In the past twenty-five years, we have lifted one billion people out of poverty and cut hunger in half!

If we compare our lives today to the lives of our ancestors a little more than two hundred years ago, the contrast is even starker. Popular period dramas tend to glorify the late pre-penicillin period of human history as a simpler time filled with happy servants, beautiful ladies, chivalrous gentlemen, and romantic carriage rides. But the truth is living conditions in the nineteenth century were pretty horrific, even if you were lucky enough to be born into the upper class. In 1800, regardless of whether you lived in a "rich" country or a "poor" one, the health conditions were so pitiable that nearly half (43 percent) of newborn children died before their fifth birthdays. Thanks to improvements in housing, sanitation, and water quality, the advent of scientific medicine, the development of low-cost vaccines, and huge leaps in agricultural productivity and nutrition, the survival of your child today is no longer a coin flip. When we fast-forward to 2015, child mortality is now down to 4.3 percent. That's ten times lower than just two hundred years ago. And due to these improvements in health and nutrition, we are also smarter and taller than our ancestors, meaning we have a greater chance not only to survive, but to thrive.

Unfortunately, our media is infatuated with reporting only the many events where things go wrong, and does not shed light on the broader, steady upward trend in global development, human health, and living conditions. We hear about incidents of violence every time we turn on the news, and yet we forget the fact that humans are now actually living in the most peaceful era in our species' history. Similarly, although we hear a lot about economic hardship and the general decline of civilization, there is an alternative, far more uplifting headline that could have just as easily and accurately been reported every day since 1990: "Despite population increases of over 2 billion since 1990, more than a billion fewer people live in poverty."[4] Of course, no such headline is ever published. As a result, two-thirds of Americans believe that the percentage of people living in extreme poverty has "almost doubled."

The magnitude of these sudden improvements in the human condition is so miraculous that it is hard to fathom. To me, it is the most striking evidence that God is moving in our time. And I believe it is the responsibility of each of us to spread this good news. Whether at the dinner table tonight, or at the grocery store, or at your church, I encourage you to tell your friends and family and neighbors about this profound evidence of God's grace and active love for humanity. This sort of rapid transformation of the human condition could not just happen on its own. It's providence. It is undoubtedly a result of great prayer.

It is also a result of decisive, bipartisan action by the US government, over many years, to provide billions of dollars in funding for humanitarian and development programs for the world's poorest, and to apply science and business practices to those programs in order to make them more effective.

We're halfway to ending hunger and poverty, and the last stretch of that difficult and righteous road now lays before us. What do we need to be doing to get there? To begin with, as active citizens living in a democratic society, we each have a critical opportunity to speak out and ensure that the United States continues to be the world's most generous funder of life-saving international humanitarian and development programs.

As Christians, we should be calling our representatives in government and reminding them of Jesus' appeal that we feed the hungry, clothe the naked, and welcome the stranger. People of faith are resilient. We are used to staying steadfast in our beliefs about what is true and good, despite others telling us they are impossible, and despite myriad challenges that sometimes cause us to falter. We need to keep advocating for programs like the President's Emergency Plan for AIDS Relief (PEPFAR) and the President's Malaria Initiative (PMI), both launched by President George W. Bush, which have saved millions of lives over the past decade. The US government's Food for Peace and Feed the Future programs feed tens of millions of people living in extreme poverty around the world each year. By investing in agriculture, resiliency, and nutrition, Feed the Future alone has lifted 23.4 million people out of poverty.

In many cases these health and development programs are implemented on the ground by Christian organizations, including large international NGOs like World Vision and Food for the Hungry, as well as much smaller faith-based organizations in Africa, South America, and Asia that are working to alleviate hunger and poverty right in their own communities. We need your voices to ensure they will have the resources they need to carry out this important work.

However, funding alone is not enough. There's a platitude that many of you who are familiar with international development have probably heard before. In fact, it's one I used to include in every stump speech. It goes something like this: "The world could end hunger and malnutrition tomorrow. All that's lacking is funding and the political will."

This is a compelling argument because it is easy. Lack of money is a surmountable challenge, and the logic of the case is simple. Hunger results from a lack of food. Money can purchase food (or drought-resistant seeds, or energy-efficient stoves—pick your input) and end hunger and undernutrition tomorrow. And it has a clear call to action—become an advocate for more nutrition funding. If everyone becomes an advocate for nutrition funding, eventually enough money will be spent, and everyone will be fed.

The issue with this argument is that it isn't correct. We lack more than the political will to end hunger. We lack knowledge. Certainly, money will be a big part of the solution, and funding and political will are necessary to ending hunger by 2030. Necessary, but not sufficient.

Take stunting, for example. When I travel to the field and meet children in areas where stunting is highly pervasive, one of the first things I do is ask them how old they are. I am often shocked by their answers. Regularly, children appear five years younger than they actually are. Their small height for their age, caused by a chronic lack of nutritious food in their first one thousand days of life, will cause them lifelong problems including stunted cognitive development, lowered lifetime earning potential, and a greater susceptibility to diseases.

On its surface, stunting seems like a problem that should be easy to solve with enough money. If children receive enough nutritious foods in the first one thousand days of their lives, they will avoid the lifelong burden of stunting. Advocates can make a compelling case for increasing nutrition funding by showing politicians some variation of this photo: two children stand next to one another. Though one is significantly smaller and younger-looking, they are actually the same age. One is stunted, one is not.

Unfortunately, even when we throw everything we know at the problem, all the Lancet-recommended interventions, fully financed and funded and scaled, the best-case result that we can expect from a four- to five-year nutrition program is a 20 percent reduction in stunting. Oftentimes it's much less. A 20 percent reduction in the number of stunted kids is still a tremendous achievement and means that standard stunting programming can still often achieve a higher return on investment than almost any other type of health or development programming in many countries. In fact, the Copenhagen Consensus recently found that across development investments, in terms of the costs and benefits of various solutions to world problems, fighting malnutrition should be the top priority.[5] However, if 20 percent reductions are the best we can expect with today's technology and approaches, that means that at least 80 percent of the stunting problem remains a mystery that we are not yet fully equipped to address.

As we fight for greater funding for nutrition, we need to acknowledge these limitations and present them as real and difficult problems. Glossing over these gaps doesn't help the cause of ending hunger. In fact, it can endanger the cause by making people take global hunger advocates less seriously. Science and politics will have to inform one another if we're going to continue making massive strides toward ending hunger in the decade ahead.

So, in addition to supporting advocacy efforts around global malnutrition, our foundation will also be investing tens of millions of dollars over the next few years to support rigorous, early-phase implementation research to identify innovative, multisectoral approaches to improve nutrition programming. Through a close working relationship with USAID and other major global nutrition funders, we will work together to gather evidence and bring the most effective and sustainable innovations to scale. Ultimately, we will find new and improved ways of delivering life-saving nutrition programming and ensure that every dollar invested in nutrition goes even further. If one dollar invested in nutrition today yields on average forty-five dollars in returns (Copenhagen Consensus), we will identify and scale the next-generation approaches that will allow one dollar to yield fifty or even one hundred dollars. In the process, we will also break down silos across the global health and development space, mobilize new domestic resource commitments, and work hand in hand with host governments to establish nutrition programming that is sustainable, bridges sectors, builds resiliency, and promotes self-reliance.

Research and advocacy are two sides of the same coin. Good advocacy should be rooted in strong evidence. On the flip side of things, you can fund all the rigorous research that you want around a breakthrough idea, and that doesn't mean anyone is going to pay attention. There are so many innovative pilot projects out there, and yet so few of them ever get funded and implemented beyond the initial pilot project. Innovation needs advocacy to be brought to scale.

If researchers want to bring innovations to scale, they need to start asking themselves the same question advocates are trained to ask the mirror each morning: How can I sell this? Our sector's advocacy experts can help researchers understand the latest data on what plays well with decision makers and the general public, and they might have great ideas on how to specifically frame projects with this in mind.

Unlike so many other major problems of our time, malnutrition is by no means intractable. We already know a great deal about what works. We have developed many types of nutrition programming that are well proven to be cost-effective, scalable, and sustainable. Our foundation has been funding this type of programming for several years now, and we have seen the results firsthand. And we have seen entire countries like Peru and Ghana double down and cut malnutrition in half in just a few years.

While finding innovations that can be applied at scale is important, it is equally critical that international efforts to eradicate hunger and malnutrition focus deeply on the specific local context in which they are working. In our work, we have found that the underlying causes of malnutrition in one village can be completely different from the underlying causes in other villages just a few miles away. An international organization is never going to be able to understand these community-specific contexts as well as the people who live in those communities. It is time that effective community-based organizations (CBOs) move from being implementing partners to taking a leading role in shaping the interventions that will be implemented in their communities. As USAID administrator Mark Green says, in international development, we should all be in the business of putting ourselves out of a job and allowing countries themselves to take the lead. We won't be able to end hunger by 2030 without understanding local contexts and empowering local organizations.

Eradicating hunger is always going to be more difficult than reducing it. We need new ideas. We need to test these ideas and make sure they are practical on a large scale in difficult contexts. Once we have rigorously tested these ideas and found them effective, we need people who will tell the world about them.

The only way we as a community will end hunger by 2030 is through a combination of groundbreaking research, interagency cooperation to apply that research at scale, empowerment of local organizations with deep knowledge of the specific local contexts that lead to hunger, and smart and tireless work from citizens like you who are willing to advocate for more resources to end hunger. Everyone has a stake in ending hunger and malnutrition, and everyone has a role to play.

In the ongoing chaos, and despite the cruelty and suffering still around us, let us hold on to the good news and dare together to follow God's wild and freeing Spirit. Let us dream dreams and see visions and put our dreams and visions of God's justice and love into action. In the past twenty-five years, our world has cut poverty, hunger, and undernutrition in half.

Onward to 2030.

NAME: Esther
AGE: 34
LOCATION: Ixcuintepec, Oaxaca, Mexico

Editors' Note: Esther is a mother of five children—four girls and a boy—ranging in age from five to sixteen years old. She lives in a tiny rural village high in the mountains of the Oaxaca region of southern Mexico, where her husband and most of their extended families are small-plot coffee growers. They are subsistence farmers—using their small plots of land that are a three-hour hike into the steep terrain of the forest from their homes in Ixcuintepec to grow just enough, in a good year, to keep their families housed, clothed, and fed for the next year.

Unfortunately, in 2018, most of the coffee crops in this region of Oaxaca were devastated by a plague of rust mold that destroyed more than 90 percent of the crops. Relief organizations such as California-based Growers First donated thousands of new coffee plants to help the coffee growers recover, but new coffee plants will not produce adequate beans for harvest for three-to-five years. Many of the coffee-growing families in this region—including Esther and her family of seven—were in dire straits. Further exacerbating an already bad situation, for more than a year, Esther has been suffering from an intestinal-digestive disorder that has left her in great pain and with a colostomy, unable to work. The day she spoke to us in August 2018, she had just made the difficult twelve-hour trip by bus from Ixcuintepec to the Growers First center in Ixtepec, where the director took her to see doctors at the local hospital.

● ● ●

There have been times in my life when food was scarce, and we weren't sure where we would get the money to pay for things. But this past year has been the very worst of my life. It's never been more difficult than it is today.

I have a very big problem—very big and difficult. I trust in God that I will find some doctors who are truly going to help me. But they've told me a lot of money will be needed for me to be well. I need a lot of your support in prayer.

Pray for me, please, so that everything turns out well when I go to the doctor. I may have to go to Monterey (more than one thousand miles north of her home) in search of better doctors to attend to me because in Oaxaca, they no longer want to.

I've gone to see doctors for a year now, suffering in bed. And my story from before I became ill is very different from today. Before, I made bread in our family bakery to feed my children. It was a happiness for all of us because I supported my husband and the coffee-growing business with selling the bread—and I was healthy.

But now that I find myself in poor health, it's a bit complicated and sad for me. I'm not able to work, and I am suffering. My children now have to work, and they have been working hard. They have been working despite us not wanting them to—they are minors. But they are making such great efforts. There are moments that I have cried to see them like this, and I cry because I am not the same person I used to be.

We now are living a complicated, very difficult life. There are moments that I get desperate and I say I no longer want to live, but I ask the Lord for strength—that God will help me and allow me to see my children grow. I trust in God.

Thank you to the Americans who have sent clothes and supplies and reinforcements. During the recent earthquake we found their support and thank God for it. We thank God for everything that has been a blessing for us.

My husband is a farmer. He dedicates himself to milpa, beans, corn, and coffee. He just planted a little bit of coffee, and the plants are growing. My oldest daughter has stepped in to help me and take over many of my tasks as mother. She had to stop her studies and stop going to school, though, to help support the family by selling bread, making tamales, and, well, helping us find our "daily bread"—which sustains us.

Please take care of your health. When you are strong and healthy and have a minor pain, make sure you go see a doctor before you end up living the kind of life I'm now living, which is very hard and very complicated.

I didn't see a doctor in time because there were none nearby and I didn't have the money to see doctors who are farther away. Now my health is complicated and life itself is very difficult.

A PATH TO PEACE
AND STABILITY

DAVID BEASLEY

After decades of progress in reducing hunger around the world, hunger is fighting back. It's on the rise because of conflict, and it will continue to rise unless we create a better path to peace and stability.

I have seen the toll of the conflict and hunger cycle up close and personal. Since I became the executive director of the United Nations World Food Programme (WFP) in April 2017, I've been to the four regions closest to famine: Yemen, South Sudan, northeast Nigeria, and Somalia—all filled with hungry people because of human-made conflict.

I've also seen the wounds on the Rohingya refugees from Myanmar. I've talked to those fleeing fighting in the Central African Republic, and people desperate to return to their small farms in the Democratic Republic of the Congo. I've visited hard-to-reach, war-torn areas of Syria and talked to Syrian refugees in Lebanon.

In all these places, I've met many people who worry about food. But nearly every time I've talked to them, they've asked for help

Some of the material in this chapter first appeared as David Beasley, "A Path to Peace and Stability Through Food Aid," *PRIO Blogs* (April 13, 2018), blogs.prio.org/2018/04/a-path-to-peace-and-stability-through-food-aid.

creating peace first. They see clearly that their food security is inextricably tied to fewer community tensions, less violent extremism, and more mutual cooperation. The rest of us should see it too—more conflict leads to more hunger, and persistent hunger also creates the kind of instability that leads to more conflict.

The number of chronically hungry people hit 815 million in 2016, up from 777 million in 2015.[1] When it comes to severe hunger—people who need emergency assistance because they have no other way to get the food they need to stay alive—we have seen an even more dramatic increase. Those numbers rose 55 percent in just two years, from eighty million in 2015 to 124 million last year.[2]

The reason for all this misery is conflict. Conflict drives ten out of the thirteen largest hunger crises in the world. Sixty percent of the world's hungry live in conflict zones—90 percent if you don't count the number of food insecure in China and India. Hunger fuels long-standing grievances and disputes over land, livestock, and other assets.

The consequences of conflict and hunger are most severe on children. Stunting, which is a condition that impairs growth in young bodies, is usually caused by hunger, malnutrition, and poor health. Seventy-five percent of the world's stunted children live in a conflict area.[3]

It should not surprise anyone to learn that 80 percent of the World Food Programme's operational budget is spent in countries where human-made conflict is present. For example, our per-day cost to feed someone in a non-conflict area is about thirty cents, but it is more than fifty cents a day in a conflict zone. Multiply that by millions, and you clearly can see that food and other humanitarian assistance is vastly more expensive when people are shooting at each other.

The vast links between food insecurity and conflict contribute to other serious issues within these nations. My friend US Senator Pat Roberts of Kansas has painted the problem in perhaps the most succinct way. He says, "Show me a nation that cannot feed itself, and I'll show you a nation in chaos."[4] Analysis from WFP's affiliate WFP-USA backs this up, showing that food insecurity produces instability, and that instability produces food insecurity.

About 80 percent of the countries that have severe food insecurity are also considered fragile—countries with governance and economic issues that make resolving the problems of conflict and hunger even more difficult. By 2030, it is predicted that as many as two-thirds of the world's poor will live in nations that can be classified as fragile.[5] It's not surprising, then, that just about every country near the bottom of the World Bank's Political Instability Index has a high degree of food insecurity and near-constant conflict within its borders.

Countries with the highest level of food insecurity coupled with armed conflict also have the highest outward migration of refugees. Our own research shows that for each 1 percent increase in hunger, there is a 2 percent increase in migration.[6] Refugees and asylum seekers are on the move because they feel they have no choice, even though none of them really wants to move. Nearly every Syrian we talked to for our 2017 study "At the Root of Exodus" said they wanted to go back to Syria when it was secure and stable at home.

This isn't surprising. People want to stay with their families, with familiar surroundings, in the place they call home. Sometimes they will stay at great risk to their own personal safety.

But sometimes there's a tipping point.

In mid-2015, asylum applications to Europe from Syria spiked from ten thousand a month to sixty thousand a month when humanitarian assistance was slashed. That, plus the conflict, prompted people to decide to take the risk and move.

From Africa, even the dangers of crossing the Mediterranean do not appear to be deterring those who flee conflict, hunger, and poor economic conditions. Data from the United Nations High

Commissioner for Refugees (UNHCR) shows that in 2016, 730,000 people from Africa were in Europe as refugees or asylum seekers. That's nearly double the 360,000 from Africa who were in Europe in 2010.

The conditions that lead to this migration-forcing instability are a wonderful breeding ground for violent extremism. It makes the extremists' recruiting efforts far too easy. As the United Nations Development Programme said in a report last year, "Where there is injustice, deprivation, and desperation, violent extremist ideologies present themselves as a challenge to the status quo and a form of escape."[7]

Sometimes, it's even simpler than that. These extremist groups sometimes present themselves as the only way to survive. One woman in Syria told our researchers, "The men had to join extremist groups to be able to feed us. It was the only option."

Perhaps the most prominent example of how a hunger crisis played into the hands of extremists came in 2011 in Somalia, where drought, a food price spike, and civil war converged in a famine that led to a quarter-million people dying.

Researchers have documented that during this time, al-Shabaab kept humanitarians from reaching hungry people with aid *and* the militant group offered the hungry money to join its ranks. One UNHCR official called the famine "a boon" for al-Shabaab's recruitment efforts.[8]

It is critical to point out that the World Food Programme is fully committed to humanitarian law and its principles. We do not take sides; we feed the hungry and vulnerable wherever they are. But when food is a weapon of war, we have to look for another way.

What we need to do is make food a weapon of peace.

Food and other forms of assistance have helped people remain in their countries despite difficult circumstances and have helped refugees return home, to earn a living and provide hope for their children.

It is crystal clear to me that effective humanitarian assistance is pro-peace. It not only helps alleviate suffering and protects civilians affected by war and conflict, but also promotes efforts that address the root causes of conflicts and the reengagement of people in productive economic activities.

Niger is a place where these types of policies are showing progress. There, the WFP is working with several partner organizations to help more than 250,000 people in about thirty-five communes, or towns, with a multisector approach that builds resilience and stability. More precisely, the programs in Niger cover land regeneration and water harvesting, working with women's groups to plant tree nurseries and community gardens, and providing school meals through community gardens.

A concerted, focused effort such as this can create stability and the kind of conditions that help a family, a community, and a region take care of itself. That must begin with food, because nothing can happen when everyone is hungry. But it also means schools and water and roads and governance and a dozen other things.

Another key component of this pro-development, pro-peace strategy starts younger—with school children. This program is enormously cost-effective—on average, the WFP spends fifty dollars to feed a child in school *for an entire year.* And for some parents, that food is the reason they send their child to school, because they're assured their child will get at least one meal that day.

But the program does more than that. Children sit down, and talk, and laugh together while eating, and I believe that time helps these children see each other as people. The meal binds them together. And when they're older, those bonds are harder to break.

That's what Hatem Ben Salem, the minister of education in Tunisia, told me this year as he reflected on his "warm memory" of his experiences with school meals as a child. "Lunchtime at school offered an opportunity for children from diverse backgrounds, rich and poor, to sit around a table and share a hot meal," he wrote.

Military spending around the world is now at roughly 2 trillion dollars a year.[9] But the programs highlighted here could save us some of that money. Or, as US Secretary of Defense James Mattis has said, effective humanitarian assistance means he needs to buy fewer bullets.[10] So, working toward the global goal of zero hunger truly is the best defense for the nations of the world, because it creates stability that reduces the risk of conflict.

That stability is the kind of world that Fazle, a man I met in Pakistan in the spring of 2018, lives in now. Constant war drove him, his wife, and their four children away from their home and farm eight years earlier. They loved their home, but with all the shooting and armed extremist groups, Fazle and his family had to leave or endure the death, destruction, and instability that comes with war.

But seven years later, Fazle and his family returned home, and are doing well. They received six months of food aid from the World Food Programme and the Pakistan government, giving them a cushion that allowed them, in turn, to get into a program with the UN Food and Agriculture Organization that helped Fazle set up a nursery. Now he's earning about 130 dollars a month, four times his previous income.

Fazle and his family want to live, work, and pursue their dreams. Food security was the cornerstone on which the rest of their new start was built—not just saving lives, but changing them.

8

BRINGING EVERYONE TO THE TABLE

HELENE GAYLE

Instability—whether it's human-made or the result of natural disasters, conflicts, or poor governance—is a major reason why some people and countries are able to move forward, and others are not.

Nutrition is the fulcrum for both good health and strong economies. It is a core, basic need for all people—the one factor that has a huge impact on all other areas of life and almost every challenge facing the world today. If you're not healthy and you don't have access to education, it's also difficult to get an economic foothold.

And yet, in all my years working in global health and international development, I've never seen an adequate focus on nutrition.

Nutrition is not a sexy issue. It's not glitzy, and it's not the new disease in town. It doesn't have some of the eye-catching qualities of health issues that unfold more dramatically. It's not Ebola or the Zika virus.

Malnutrition and hunger have been around for a long time. Perhaps they don't capture the imagination because they have been longstanding problems.

We know that adequate nutrition for a woman who is pregnant is a huge determiner—not only for her health, but also for the health of her child. Nutrition in the first one thousand days is essential for adequate brain and body development for young children. The importance of proper nutrition in giving children a healthy start cannot be overstated. We know that a child who goes to school hungry is not going to be able to learn. Poor nutrition often is a cause for poor educational attainment. There are so many steps along the way in which nutrition is critical to whether someone can develop appropriately, take advantage of educational opportunities, and be a strong worker in the work force.

•   •   •

Similarly, in the fight against HIV/AIDS, we have witnessed how crucial nutrition is to combating disease. We found that antiretrovirals helped with the infection, but they also allowed people to become—*if* they had adequate nutrition—healthy again. They were mutually reinforcing: antiretrovirals helped people with their overall health and status, and nutrition was a key component to antiretrovirals being effective. Because wasting was a troubling component of HIV and AIDS in the early days, before there were effective antiretroviral therapies, it was incredibly important to make sure that people living with the virus were able to maintain adequate nutrition.

Since President George W. Bush launched the President's Emergency Plan for AIDS Relief (PEPFAR) in 2003, the United States has been the largest donor to HIV programs in the world. To date, we have provided more than $80 billion in funding to combat HIV/AIDS globally. As of March 30, 2018, PEPFAR had supported life-saving antiretroviral treatment for more than fourteen million people—including more than one million children—saving the lives of millions. In its first fifteen years, PEPFAR enabled more than 2.2 million children to be born HIV-free, allowed 85.5 million people to be tested for HIV/AIDS, and provided support for 6.4 million orphans, vulnerable children, and their caregivers worldwide.

It is with good cause that PEPFAR is heralded as one of the most effective and efficient US foreign assistance programs in the nation's history. The US budget for fiscal year 2018 allocated $4.65 billion for PEPFAR. Yet, the total budget for USAID and US State Department nutrition programs was $125 million for FY18. We aren't spending enough in nutrition. But we also are in a world of unlimited resources.

INNOVATION IS KEY

Sometimes I think the money itself is not the issue as much as how we use it. Are we making sure that the money we are spending is as effective as possible? More important is thinking about how we approach nutrition in new ways.

Are we doing enough on the agricultural front? Are we doing enough with the business and the private sector? Agribusiness? Are there companies that could look for innovative ways to make sure that we can get the most from the nutrition that is available?

It's not just about aid for nutrition, it's also about what we are doing to increase agricultural productivity so that countries can be agriculturally productive and have the resources internally to provide for their citizens.

There are a lot of ways we could come together and use the resources we have more effectively. Yes, I'd love to see our nutrition dollars doubled or tripled. But we need to make sure we are thinking about the most effective ways of spending the resources we have.

What are the right kinds of partnerships with the public sector, the private sector, and the not-for-profit sector? How might we be able to look at both nutrition itself and how we get adequate nutrition to populations?

The agriculture nexus is extremely important to keep in mind. Nutrition is linked to agriculture, which in many societies is the biggest economic engine and where many people make their livelihood.

INTEGRATION IS ESSENTIAL

How do we look at new technologies and innovation, particularly in agriculture? A lot of work has been done in recent years around food fortification—micronutrient fortification of locally-grown foods so that they have the highest nutritional content possible—and new ways of looking at increasing crop yields.

Programs such as the Alliance for a Green Revolution in Africa (AGRA), for instance, which is funded through a partnership between the Rockefeller Foundation and the Bill & Melinda Gates Foundation, looked at the best ways to increase agricultural productivity and helped create the sense of a new green revolution in Africa. There are a lot of efforts like this one that explore the integration of nutrition and agriculture.

From the services side of the equation, we need to look at how we ensure that nutrition is integrated, particularly among the most vulnerable populations. Integrating nutrition into child health services, so that children coming through for their routine immunizations also receive nutritional support, is another innovative approach that's gained momentum. The same is true for pregnant women and antenatal services.

Gender also is a key factor in nutrition, food security, and overall hunger. There's a huge need to make sure the nutrition of girls and women is prioritized. In many places throughout the world, women and girls are the last to be fed in a family. Men and boys are fed preferentially—and women and girls get whatever is left over.

There are cultural shifts that need to take place. Families and whole societies need to change the way they think about the importance of nutrition for women and girls, being attentive particularly to the nutritional needs of pregnant and lactating women.

We also need to think about how such shifts get integrated into schools and educational facilities, where nutrition can be taught to children so they understand its value. It's especially important for girls as they become adolescents and their nutritional needs change.

When it comes to ensuring that men and boys start appreciating the need for all members of their family to have access to adequate nutrition, there is an educational component, and there is a health care and health services component. They must be integrated.

A BETTER STRATEGY

One of the Sustainable Development Goals put forth by the United Nations is to end global hunger by 2030. It's a lofty goal, and we have fewer than a dozen years to accomplish it.

I believe it is totally possible, *if* we put the right kind of resources and priority toward the issue.

We know there is enough food to feed everybody on the planet. The problem is not the lack of resources; it's that they are maldistributed. This gets at one of the most crucial questions to answer about global hunger: Are we making sure that food gets to where it's needed most?

I live in a country where the biggest problem is food wastage. Even in the United States, we aren't getting food to the people who need it most, who are suffering from a lack of access to healthy, nutritious food.

We have a lot of work to do in terms of food distribution in addition to enacting some of the strategies that could help increase food yield and make it more accessible. We must start by getting everyone to the table to address the issues, and then we must have a clear strategy for doing the work.

But the big issue is having a clear, doable set of targeted goals that people all can rally behind, goals that coordinate different people's roles. In other words, if, say, I'm in agribusiness, how will my task be different from if I were a health service provider?

Having a plan that maps out the goals we're trying to reach is great, but what is my part in it and what is yours? Everybody ought to understand what they should bring to the table in order to be able to accomplish something in a coordinated way.

My hope is that global hunger—nutrition, food security, and other related issues—is something that people will start rallying around. I hope we realize that, if we're going to achieve some of the Sustainable Development Goals, nutrition needs to be very, very high on the agenda.

Everybody looks for a magic bullet. But it doesn't exist.

Ending global hunger is about doing what we know works, doing it consistently, and doing it for the long haul.

WHAT TO DO ABOUT MALNOURISHED PEOPLE AROUND THE WORLD

TONY CAMPOLO

I try to comprehend all of the ramifications of having millions and millions of children around the world grow up without the food they need to nourish their bodies. What I do know comes from what I have seen and heard during my travels in poor countries such as Haiti and Mali.

I have seen children whose growth was stunted because they were underfed during their crucial early childhood years. Their growth was hindered because of diet, and it was impossible to guess their ages. Boys and girls that were eleven and twelve years of age appeared to be seven or eight. Such children are easy to spot, because often their hair has turned the color of rust from lack of protein and iron in their diets. At first, they seemed well behaved as I watched them sitting motionless in the church services where I preached, but later I learned their stillness was the result of being too weak to move.

I have heard from teachers in these countries who face the problem of children whose brains are so inadequately developed because of nutritional deficiencies that they have trouble learning. These teachers were convinced that there were students who could not keep up in their learning with other children their age, not because of any birth defects, but because they were suffering the effects of long-term malnutrition. Teachers told me stories of children who have fallen asleep in class because they were too weak to pay attention to the lessons of the day.

Facing the painful dilemmas created by inadequate diets creates challenges that can be daunting. In our endeavors to address the problems related to poor nutrition, we must face the sad and easily overlooked reality that much of the food produced in poor countries is never eaten. To get to market, many farmers have to transport their produce on wooden carts over poor, bumpy roads, leading to the vegetables and fruits arriving damaged and spoiled. Even if the farmers do get their products safely to market, they sometimes find there are few buyers. The people who need the nutritious produce the farmers offer would love to buy it, but lack the funds to purchase what is for sale.

Visitors to marketplaces in poor countries surely have seen this unfortunate situation. They might observe piles of unsold food that have stood out under the heat of the sun all day long and rotted. It is sad to watch this once edible food being swept up and carted away to a garbage dump. And yet there are ways of addressing these problems that could rescue the farmers' endangered produce and avoid this waste.

Several years ago, one of my students traveled to Sudan as a missionary under the auspices of the Sudan Interior Missions. He had the means and knew how to set up a very simple food-processing plant back in the hills of Sudan where some hard-working farmers were facing the problems I have just been describing. Using simple, very low-tech equipment supplied by the Ball Corporation in Muncie, Indiana, and with the guidance that company provided, he set up a micro business in which the food grown by local farmers was processed and preserved in glass jars produced by the Ball Corporation.

It didn't take long for the farmers in his vicinity to take advantage of this processing plant. With the food they had grown (especially tomatoes) preserved in glass jars, they could safely transport their produce to the market and not have to worry about spoilage if it were not sold on market day. The preserved food could be taken back to the farmers' villages and carried back to market to be put for sale again the following week. The jars of food also could be taken for sale at other markets some distance away without the processed fruits and vegetables going bad.

Learning of the success of the food-processing plant in Sudan, some of us at Eastern University decided it would be a good idea to set up a graduate program to train and equip missionary entrepreneurs to go to developing countries and start micro businesses and micro industries that could provide employment for indigenous peoples. Now, more than thirty-five years later, our Eastern University graduates have lived out that vision, and it has been estimated by former university president David Black that they have generated a quarter of a million jobs among very needy people in developing countries.

In South Africa, Eastern graduates have started programs manufacturing clothing, which are sold on the world market as well as locally. In Haiti, they have produced toys, which are sold throughout Europe via a distribution company in Holland. The list of enterprises is long and what these unique missionaries have done is inspiring, to say the least.

Our graduates encourage indigenous people to become entrepreneurs, so that when their businesses succeed these people can say, "We did it ourselves!"

It does not require super intelligence to figure out that when poor people in developing nations earn money, they are likely to spend that money on food, especially for their children. The businesses we are developing help to provide good nutrition for their families.

As important as micro businesses are in helping poor people gain the financial resources essential to properly feed their children, it is equally important that people of good will collectively address the problems that rich and powerful countries have created for poor people in Third World countries.

There are policy changes that must be made, especially when it comes to trade relations between countries. One particular concern has to do with what is defined as "free trade." The policy of free trade seems like something that those who espouse democratic capitalism should applaud. It sounds like a good thing to eliminate taxes for goods coming into the United States from poor countries, and for the goods we ship into those poor countries also to be tax free.

Indeed, this does sound good until we learn that American farmers are subsidized to the tune of billions of dollars each year. That means that American farmers are able to ship their subsidized wheat to a poor country such as Haiti and put it on the market for a price that is lower than that of the wheat produced by Haitian farmers. This situation drives many Haitian farmers out of business.

President Bill Clinton was one of a succession of American presidents who advocated the free trade policies just described. He said before a congressional committee exploring ways to help Haiti in the aftermath of the horrendous earthquake a few years ago, "It [the free trade policy] may have been good for some of my farmers in Arkansas, but it has not worked [for the farms in Haiti]."[1]

This short essay does not allow for a full explanation of all the economic policy changes that must be made on the macro level by government action, but hopefully it will create a sense that policy changes are necessary if we are to address the problem of malnutrition in the poor countries of the world. Consider how problems of global warming and climate change, which can be addressed only by the actions of government, are affecting food production. It doesn't take rocket science to figure out how incentives to save the planet from an ecological disaster must be executed if we are to address the massive needs of malnourished people.

•   •   •

There is one overarching problem we must solve: we must avert wars. Wars destroy the ability of people to grow food. Fields of grain are wiped out by advancing armies. Food supplies that could feed the hungry are diverted and stolen to feed the armies. Most importantly, wars cause farmers to give up growing food because they sense that it is all to no avail. Wars create hunger, and unless we are committed to stopping wars, the peace necessary to end hunger and malnutrition will continue to be only a distant hope.

We can make a difference in addressing the tragic malnutrition of so many people in poor countries, but that will require important initiatives on both the micro level with small entrepreneurship ventures as well as government action on the macro level.

This essay only hints at some of the many things that can and should be done to properly feed the poor of the world. We must do all we can to let it be known that the impoverished people of the world are not likely to remain passive while their children suffer from malnutrition.

What is needed is a commitment by the great nations of the world to develop and execute a plan to bring about changes on both the micro level and the macro level. By calling for such cooperation, the religious people of the world can exercise their influence to require all the leaders of the world to do what needs to be done to end hunger.

True religion is able to stir the hearts and minds of people to reach out to the poor and oppressed. It might even motivate world governments toward compassion and away from lesser concerns. At the base of each of the world's great religions is a call to feed the hungry, and it is with this call that we could and should begin.

"REMEMBER US WHEN YOU COME INTO YOUR KINGDOM"

Hunger in America

JEREMY K. EVERETT

In 2014, US Congress established the National Commission on Hunger, a bipartisan, ten-member commission created to find ways the United States could more effectively and efficiently address the issue of hunger. I was lucky enough to be appointed to the commission.

In order to best understand the issue, the commission traveled to communities throughout the country to hear directly from the people. One trip took us to the American Southwest, where we visited tribal lands in southern New Mexico and desert communities along the Texas-Mexico border. The trip was in the early summer, the desert sun was already hot, and traveling across the region on a small tour bus was exhausting. We went from community to community, listening to the stories of individual people, groups, and organizations committed to addressing the food needs of their communities in creative ways. We heard heartbreaking stories of hunger and poverty, and the spiraling effects of both on families struggling simply to make enough money to get by each week.

The end of our trip took us into the city of El Paso, Texas, directly on the border with Mexico, where we sat down with a group of elders from the community on one of our last site visits. The elder women and men had become acquainted some time earlier in a citizenship class they were taking at the La Fe Community Center in downtown El Paso. Most of them had lived in the United States their entire lives and had raised their children—many of whom enlisted in the US military and were serving on active duty in the Middle East—for their adopted country.

These undocumented elders were neither rapists nor drug smugglers. They were business owners, welders, mechanics, field laborers, custodians, and hotel housekeepers, mothers and fathers and grandparents. They shared a collective wish to die as citizens of the nation where they had reared their families and spent the bulk of their lives. They also had something else in common: each regularly experienced hunger.

Our conversation lasted a little over an hour. Before we went our separate ways, I asked them pointedly, "Do you have any food to eat?" Hearing this question, one proud, elderly man with a chiseled chin and a pointed mustache, wordlessly buried his head in his hands and began to weep. His wife sat up, straightened her dress, and then spoke: "Occasionally we are able to put food on the table. When we do, it is normally one meal a day. I will make us a plate of beans and a couple of tortillas. . . . We are older so we don't need as much."

Her comments seemed to resound with the group of elders. At that point one of the men looked up, wiped his tears, and said, "Remember us when you come into your kingdom."[1]

Overcome, I quickly excused myself, hurried down an empty hallway, pushed my way through the bathroom door, and wept.

•   •   •

My home congregation in Texas regularly sings a Taizé chant that repeats the words of the thief who was crucified on the cross next to Jesus, who asks the dying son of God, "Jesus, remember me when you come into your kingdom. Jesus, remember me when you come into your kingdom." We sing it over and over and over again. But it wasn't until I heard the words pronounced by that wise, humble Mexican elder that I realized, compared to many of our neighbors around the globe, I already was living in a kingdom. Before that moment, I had thought about the "kingdom" the thief on the cross mentioned only as it related to Jesus, and creating the kingdom of heaven on earth sometime in the future. The Mexican elder took those familiar words and flipped them, revealing a perspective that was new to me. After all, he was preparing to leave our conversation and return to his home, not enough food, and the isolation many elderly people in our nation experience every day, while I would return to my comfy hotel room and an ample meal before heading to the halls of power in Washington, DC, to deliver our report.

"Remember us when you come into your kingdom."

The following day, we stumbled out of our bus and were rushed into the La Fe Community Center to hear public testimony. There in the large, empty auditorium, we took our seats at a row of tables on an elevated platform facing the audience. The arrangement unfortunately meant that we were physically looking down at the people who stood before us to share their stories, as if they were testifying before a panel of judges. The room soon began to fill, and we called on the first of over a dozen people invited to give their testimonies. The public forum was scheduled to last for ten hours and include several hours of testimonies from people who had been invited to speak, followed by several more hours of testimony from anyone who wanted to have their voice heard.

Quite a few hours later, Dr. Joe Sharkey, a professor and public health expert specializing in food insecurity among underserved populations, who was leading a research project in the *colonias* communities along the Mexican border, took his seat at the table to share his experiences of addressing hunger and health issues. He began with the story of one of his public health workers, Linda, and her visit to homes in the *colonias*.

If you're not familiar with *colonias*, it may be difficult for you to grasp the living conditions that they present. These particular *colonias* in west Texas sit on the far edges of urban areas and sprawl into the desert. Often, they have neither running water nor electricity, much less paved roads. Homes in the *colonias* tend to be built with the materials at hand, and it is not uncommon to see a single room home with one wall made of corrugated metal, another of plywood, and another of rocks salvaged from the surrounding land. The property on which the homes sit in the *colonias* typically is not owned by the residents themselves, but rather is leased from landowners who may come take it back whenever they please. We do not often think of people in the United States living in conditions such as these, but in the *colonias* of rural border towns, populated largely by Mexican-American and Mexican immigrant communities, they are the status quo.

Dr. Sharkey explained to us that public health workers such as Linda used a simple set of questions to assess the health and well-being of the residents they visited. While checking on Maria, a patient who lived in a *colonia* that occasionally had electricity, Linda began asking the usual survey questions about the health of Maria's family. For her final question Linda asked, "Maria, do you have any food in the house?"

"Hearing the question," Dr. Sharkey recalled, "Maria's head slowly lowered under the weight of shame and guilt." His description of her reaction was sadly similar to the reactions of the elders when I'd asked them something similar the previous day. Without saying a word, Maria guided Linda to her kitchen and pointed to a small refrigerator. Linda opened it and saw that it was completely empty but for a small bag of chicken bones. Puzzled, Linda asked Maria, "Why is there a bag of chicken bones inside your fridge?" Through tears, Maria said, "So when my children open the refrigerator door they will at least see that something is there."

In my work in Texas, I have visited many homes in *colonias* across the border region. I have met many mothers like Maria and interacted with many of their children living in similar situations. Listening to Dr. Sharkey tell stories that mirrored my experiences in the region, I couldn't help thinking, *We can do better than this.*

Congress sent our commission throughout the country to try to identify the root causes of hunger, and what we can do as a nation to improve lives. What we discovered was hardly a surprise: for most people, food insecurity (a lack of access to food) was the direct result of economic insecurity (a lack of funds). But economic insecurity— why they didn't have enough money—was contextual. For the residents of the desert *colonias* along the Mexican border, it was their lack of legal status as citizens that resulted in low-paying jobs that kept them food insecure.

"Remember us when you come into your kingdom."

UNDERSTANDING U.S. HUNGER

So, who is experiencing hunger in the United States and why? In our nation, some populations bear the burdens of poverty and hunger more than others. They include senior adults, single-parent families with young children,[2] people with disabilities,[3] Native Americans,[4] people with family members who are incarcerated,[5] immigrants,[6] people experiencing declines in mental and physical health,[7, 8] and minority households.[9]

Presently in the United States, 40.6 million people live in poverty.[10] Of those, 13.3 million are children, and 4.6 million are senior adults.[11] More than forty-one million Americans are considered food insecure, and 6.5 million children live in food-insecure households.[12] Moreover, every county in the United States has reported food insecurity among a percentage of its populations.[13]

The term *food insecure* is the technical term we use when describing hunger. It is defined as "a lack of access to enough healthy food to live a healthy lifestyle."[14] When I served on the commission we used the term *very low food security*—meaning someone whose food intake is reduced because of the lack of resources for food—interchangeably with the word *hunger*.[15]

In the United States, hunger is primarily episodic, meaning people who experience hunger may not experience it daily.[16] Exhausted food budgets are more commonly seen at the end of the month, and may be a predictor of further health inequities.[17]

There are a variety of reasons why people in the United States experience hunger. The first and most prevalent is underemployment. Basically, this means that many people who experience hunger are employed, but their jobs don't pay enough to cover all of their living expenses—even when they're working multiple jobs trying to make ends meet. In San Antonio, for instance, our neighbors often would find minimum wage jobs in the hospitality industry, servicing restaurants and hotels that catered to tourists on vacation. They would supplement those jobs with additional jobs at a fast food restaurant, convenience store, or anything else they could find.

The rise of the global economy has made it cheaper to manufacture most of what we wear, drive, plug in, and even eat outside of the United States. So, for America's poor, finding gainful employment has become increasingly difficult.

A second reason why people experience hunger in our nation is tied directly to educational achievement. Simply put, to avoid hunger and poverty in twenty-first-century America, you must graduate from high school and also earn an additional degree, regardless of whether it's from a technical school, a two-year associate's program, or a four-year college or university. In our current economic climate, without a degree from an institution of higher learning, it's virtually impossible to secure employment that pays a living wage.

Poverty, hunger, and a lack of education quickly can become a vicious cycle. A person needs to have an education in order to have the best chance of not living in poverty and, therefore, with food insecurity and hunger. But living in poverty is a detriment to getting an education. In fact, some of the most important predictors for whether a student will graduate from high school are reading at a third-grade level or below, family poverty, family structure, and concentrated poverty at the neighborhood level.[18] Hunger often contributes to higher school dropout rates, grade repetition, and special education.[19] There are always exceptions, but if you are not the exception your chances of living in poverty and experiencing hunger increase dramatically with a lack of educational attainment.

Family structure can be another reason people experience hunger in the United States. Being a single parent with a full-time job must be an incredibly tough prospect. Who takes the kids to school? You do. Who makes dinner? You do. Who works all day to pay for everything they need and what you need and then some? You do. Add to that the desire many single parents have to improve the family's economic condition by going back to school. You might have to be superhuman to manage it all.

The hunger rate among households headed by a single mother is four times that of households headed by a married couple and twice that of households headed by a single father.[20] Naturally, households with a single wage earner are likely to earn less than households with two wage earners, which only magnifies difficulties for those living in impoverished households—particularly women, who currently earn just 82 percent of what their male counterparts do.[21]

Race, ethnicity, and gender also influence who experiences hunger and how. In the United States, people of color are more likely to experience hunger than Caucasians are.[22] Whether we want to admit it, the wounds of racism in our nation have not been healed. We have had our moments of triage such as the abolition of slavery and the Civil Rights Movement of the 1960s, which were critical steps to stop the hemorrhaging of racism's hatred, bigotry, and indifference that pervade our history. But we have not taken sufficient steps toward true healing on a national level. We did not honor our commitment to reparations or create and convene a Truth and Reconciliation Commission the way post-Apartheid South Africa did. We have not integrated our neighborhoods, churches, or social groups. As a result, people in minority households are more likely to experience poverty, food insecurity, and hunger than white households.

Other key factors that contribute toward the likelihood of experiencing poverty and hunger include exposure to violence, immigration status, housing stability, incarceration, and medical debt. Yes, there is the problem of the people whose refusal to be personally responsible for themselves leads them into poverty and hunger, but it is a much less widespread problem than we have been led to believe. From my two decades of living and working in impoverished communities, I can affirm that these folks do exist, but they are the exception, not the rule.

•   •   •

What is consistent for people experiencing hunger is that they are forced to make tradeoffs each month—deciding whether to pay their rent, medical bills, a car payment, childcare costs, electricity bill, or to buy food. Sadly, food often is the one negotiable item on their long list of financial obligations. If they don't pay the electric bill, the power is cut off. If they don't pay rent, they can be evicted. If they miss payments on the car, it will be repossessed. But, if they don't buy food, they reason, they'll just be hungry.

Sure, being hungry means being less productive at work and school, an increased risk of mental health problems, and feelings of shame, but at least they keep their home. When faced with impossible choices, people make desperate tradeoffs just to get by.

If it is true that we all are created in the image of God, then we have more in common with each other than we realize. When we identify this commonality, it becomes much easier to join in collaborative efforts to strengthen impoverished households that not only improve lives but build trust. Unfortunately, at a time of unrest in our nation and around the world, at the moment when we most need our leaders to come together for the common good, our society is more fragmented than any time since the Civil Rights era, which practically ensures the systemic problems of domestic hunger and poverty will persist.

Although our world continues toward a contentious divide, we as people of faith can take solace that, as Dr. Martin Luther King prophetically proclaimed, "The arc of a moral universe is long, but it bends towards justice."

If the Bible is correct, we will be judged, as a nation and a world, not by how we improve the quality of life for those of us who already have much, but by how we treat the hungry and the poor, the sick and the homeless—the "least of these" among us. Sacred Scripture and history repeat this claim over and over, and we must listen, not to the populist uprising, but what is underneath it. We must hear the desperation in the voices that cry out from the fringes and the margins here at home and all over our world, voices shouting for help, whether they belong to Syrian refugees, children fleeing violence in El Salvador, or the working poor in Detroit, San Angelo, or on the west side of San Antonio.

This is the kingdom of God that Christ calls us to. This is our task as people of faith.

I believe most of us want children to have ample access to food and adults to be able to find work that can sustain a family. I also imagine most of us believe that the means toward these ends do not have to pit us against each other. There seems to be a collective intuition that working together to solve our country's and the world's greatest woes is a better path forward than the mean-spiritedness and vitriol we hear from our politicians, pundits, preachers, and countless posts on social media.

Let's work together across our ideological divides, cultivating trust that will put our nation on a path toward economic opportunity for all people.

In so doing, together, we will repent for our collective scapegoating, indifference, and lack of trust in God when we, too, find ourselves in the desert. Together we will put flesh on the words of Jesus, "For I was hungry and you gave me something to eat" (Matthew 25:35).

And together, we will remember the brothers and sisters we have forsaken too long as outcasts in our kingdoms.

CAUGHT IN CONFLICT

KIMBERLY FLOWERS

Conflict and human-made disasters are the biggest cause of hunger in the world today. Currently, nearly 500 million of the 815 million people suffering from hunger live in a war-torn country.[1] These people are not part of a coalition, insurgency, or military—they are innocent civilians caught in conflict. According to the Food and Agriculture Organization of the United Nations, conflict is the main driver of food insecurity in eighteen countries and is the primary reason for the world's worst cases of hunger.[2] Studies also show causal pathways in the reverse direction—food insecurity itself can lead to unrest and political instability, particularly when rising food prices combine with a distrust in national government. Either way, the cycle needs to be broken. Four countries dealing with longstanding wars are also on the brink of famine: Yemen, Nigeria, South Sudan, and Somalia. Yemen is suffering from the world's largest cholera outbreak, restricted humanitarian access, and a complete breakdown of both basic government services and its broader economy. There are now more than twenty-two million people, or three-quarters of the population, who need humanitarian aid and protection.[3] (Imagine the *entire* population of Florida in need of emergency assistance.)

In South Sudan, armed clashes have caused farmers to abandon fertile lands, disrupted basic market flows, and spurred Africa's largest refugee crises. There are estimates that 59 percent of the population, including more than one million children are suffering from severe food insecurity.[4]

More than one million South Sudanese children did not have enough food in 2018. That bears repeating.

The situations in Yemen and South Sudan are unacceptable when we have the knowledge to prevent these tragedies and the technology to grow enough food to feed everyone on the planet. We have a humanitarian system that can save lives and rebuild communities, development interventions that can boost agricultural growth and prevent malnutrition, and political options to ensure that access to the most vulnerable is not blocked.

Famine is completely preventable in the twenty-first century.

The United States funds a network of experts to track and warn us about food crises in the hardest hit countries. They use satellite imagery, follow weather patterns, and analyze market data, among other tools, to predict the number of people who will require food assistance for the next six months. The international community uses these warnings to respond to crises around the world before they escalate. In South Sudan, which declared famine in two regions for a few months of 2017, intervention from the global community was key to preventing the situation from deteriorating. We need to scale up attention and funding, though, to meet the unprecedented humanitarian needs of 2018.

"Food is the moral right of all who are born unto this world," said Dr. Norman Borlaug,[5] who won the Nobel Peace Prize for saving an estimated one billion lives through his groundbreaking work in agriculture. Most would agree with him. Yet food is consistently used as a weapon of war.[6] It is a powerful political commodity that can entice young recruits to join a terrorist group or be used to control isolated communities. Terrorist groups such as Boko Haram in Nigeria and

Al-Shabab in Somalia exacerbate food insecurity and undermine aid efforts by controlling food aid and forcing farmers to flee from their lands, among other tactics.

These wars and the food crises they cause are particularly disconcerting when we consider the plight of hungry children. The cognitive damage a child suffers when deprived of the right blend of vitamins and minerals in the first one thousand days of life is *irreversible*. The negative consequences of chronic malnutrition are even greater when considering the compromising effects on future school and work performance.

● ● ●

If we want to end hunger, we need to tackle its root causes. The volatility of fragile states creates an environment in which vulnerable men, women, and children lack the means to survive. Severe food insecurity is ultimately driven by political decisions, which means we need more than humanitarian and development interventions. Political solutions are critical to resolve conflicts and create peace.

As a respected global leader, the United States and its actions matter. It is therefore important that the country keeps global food security as a foreign affairs priority. This includes fostering strong diplomatic relations, implementing effective international development programs, and coordinating across government agencies to leverage our assets. Addressing global hunger and malnutrition demonstrates our American values and protects our national security. US policymakers understand this well. Senator Marco Rubio has said that "foreign aid is important. If it's done right, it spreads America's influence around the world in a positive way."[7]

Republicans and Democrats agree that the economic and political stability of other countries is in our best interests, which is why they passed a bipartisan bill in 2016 called the Global Food Security Act. The legislation, which was reauthorized in September 2018, prioritizes addressing hunger, poverty, and malnutrition in developing countries. The United States reducing global hunger is supported by both sides of the political aisle because the results speak for themselves. Agricultural and nutrition development programs, funded by US tax dollars, have lifted nine million people above the poverty line and helped farmers generate 10.5 billion dollars in new agricultural sales.[8]

I have seen firsthand how development can improve the lives of those less fortunate, particularly among smallholder farmers and their families. Through research trips and congressional delegations, I have had the honor of talking with people around the world—in countries as diverse as Senegal, Guatemala, and Bangladesh—to better understand their challenges with poverty, hunger, and malnutrition and their perceptions of what types of development programming work best.

In Tanzania, I remember a proud grandmother introducing me to her healthy "one thousand days" grandbaby, explaining how incorporating a more diverse diet, including leafy vegetables and protein, significantly improved the child's health. In Ghana, I met female farmers who could grow crops year-round thanks to access to finance, better seeds, and water-saving technologies.

Since most of the world's poor (80 percent) live in rural areas and depend on farming for a living, one of the most effective ways to address poverty and hunger is through agricultural development.[9] This is why approximately 1 billion in American tax dollars has been allocated to this sector each year since 2010 through Feed the Future. It is money well spent. International development programs funded by the United States teach better agricultural practices, improve market systems, foster a better regulatory environment, and improve access to finance and quality seeds. Farmers' incomes have significantly increased—quadrupled in some cases—meaning there is extra money for children's school fees, health care, and farm equipment and supplies. This kind of programming also creates economic stability in the market and growth in the national economy—important factors when it comes to reducing both conflict and poverty alike.

Life-saving humanitarian efforts are often the first step in responding to fragile countries that don't have the kind of stability needed for investments in long-term agricultural growth. The United States has long been the global leader in providing humanitarian relief to the world's latest crises, including emergency food assistance to the most vulnerable. Last year, US food aid reached nearly seventy million people in fifty-three countries—an impressive and important feat.

Beyond the Global Food Security Act, mentioned above, Congress is considering other pieces of legislation that have a direct impact on people facing food insecurity. The Farm Bill provides international food aid though a program called Food for Peace and is also currently up for reauthorization. The newly introduced, bipartisan Food Aid Modernization Act promises greater efficiencies within Food for Peace programming, which could make our food aid programs more flexible while saving the United States money, while reaching a greater number of people in need at the same time.

Is ending hunger possible? Not unless we address its root causes, including conflict. Immediate humanitarian assistance and longer-term development programs that improve nutrition and lift people out of poverty will remain critical as complementary short- and long-term solutions. Sustainable progress, though, requires stable governments and peaceful societies that are committed to ensuring that no one goes hungry.

THE POSSIBLE IMPOSSIBLE DREAM

GABE SALGUERO

I've sung it at least a thousand times: *To dream the impossible dream. To fight the unbeatable foe. . . . To right the unrightable wrong.*

Joe Darion's lyrics to "The Impossible Dream (The Quest)" from the Broadway musical *Man of La Mancha* reflect the heart of a movement fueled by moms, dads, economists, faith leaders, governments, and activists who believe the end of hunger is achievable.

For far too long, far too many of us have suffered from myopathy when it comes to ending global hunger. Our leaders have also shared this collective nearsightedness, which makes the possibility of feeding everyone who is hungry, eradicating food insecurity, and making malnutrition a thing of the past, appear to be little more than a blurry dream.

But ending hunger is no quixotic reverie. Like Cervantes's protagonist Don Quixote, a new generation of dreamers and doers must tilt against the windmills of despair and apathy, daring to see differently and reach for what once was believed to be unattainable. At its core, the movement to end hunger is a call to envision a different future for hundreds of millions of men, women, and children around the world—a future where abject hunger is a distant memory and all of God's children have the opportunity to flourish.

Inside a tiny clinic in Malawi in 2011, my eyes opened to a new vision and the possibility of a radically more hopeful future. There I watched, captivated, as a father spent all night in the clinic with his precious daughter, Julia. She was there to receive micronutrients to help counteract the devastating effects of malnutrition that had stunted her growth.

I asked the dad his name. "My name is Hector," he answered. The same name as my father. Instantly I was drawn into their story, and Hector and Julia became the prophetic voices that awakened me to a global movement that refuses to surrender to the challenges of global hunger where shortsightedness can be deadly.

I am acquainted personally with food deserts. As a child on the Jersey Shore, I made my share of mayonnaise-sandwiches-with-iced-tea lunches. And I knew, to a much lesser degree than Julia and Hector, what it meant not to have enough. For a short time, my family and I benefitted from social safety net programs such as the Supplemental Nutrition Assistance Program (SNAP), which helped us make ends meet.

Still, even as an adult, my ignorance of the global movement to combat food crises was acute. After meeting Hector and Julia, ignorance no longer was an option. They awakened me to an international movement for proper nutrition that truly is making a difference. This movement invests in life-saving nutrition in food-distressed places around the world. In the days following my visit to Malawi, Zambia, and South Africa, mothers, doctors, economists, and pastors continued to educate me about the changes that are afoot.

ADVOCACY IS A CHRISTIAN CALLING

The cost of ignoring hunger and its consequences for the futures of women, children, families, and even entire countries requires our immediate attention. No doubt the challenges are formidable, and the work ahead is arduous. But such is our calling as believers.

Some people have asked me as an evangelical pastor, "What can the church do?" I am convinced that the gospel calls us to fight for a better future with hope and courage. Scripture entreats us not just to feed the hungry, but also to advocate actively for the poor and needy. Proverbs 31:9 says, "Speak up and judge fairly; /defend the rights of the poor and needy."

The church is not simply a direct service provider with soup kitchens, feeding programs, and global missions. We also are asked to respond to Christ's call by ensuring that no one goes (or is sent away) hungry. Jesus made it plain: "They do not need to go away. You give them something to eat" (Matthew 14:16). The church is a prophetic voice calling for laws that provide for those whom Jesus called "the least of these."

Congregations across the country are reorienting their vision and looking toward Capitol Hill. Growing numbers of Christians are aware that the church can save more lives by advocating for hungry people than by solely focusing on ministries of mercy. The clinic where Julia received treatment to combat malnutrition, for instance, is the product of faith-based non-governmental organizations (NGOs) and social entrepreneurs who dared to invest in the families and children of Malawi.

In the Hispanic evangelical congregations the National Latino Evangelical Coalition (NALEC) serves, we are adding to our compassionate ministry and global missions' foci advocacy for policies that save the lives of women and children. Churches play a key role as allies for hungry people in the corridors of power and policymaking. To be clear, this shift in our collective vision requires that we revisit how American evangelicals historically have viewed hunger and the ministry of advocacy.

As an evangelical and pastor of evangelicals, I am aware of the complicated legacy we have in dealing with hunger. Evangelical churches in the United States were at the forefront of supporting

President George W. Bush's PEPFAR initiative and other development programs around the world. In addition, our congregations have been vanguards in developing food pantries, soup kitchens, and feeding programs domestically.

There is much to celebrate in the work of evangelical congregations. Nevertheless, it is increasingly clear that more needs to be done. Congregational service without international policies that support aid for the hungry is another symptom of shortsightedness.

I can't recall the number of times I've heard preachers misinterpret Jesus' declaration, "The poor you will always have with you" (Matthew 26:11). In citing Deuteronomy, Jesus is referencing a text that concludes with a national moral imperative toward generosity. In Deuteronomy 15:11, after reminding the nation of the presence of the poor, God demands, "I command you to be openhanded toward your fellow Israelites who are poor and needy in your land." Jesus' reminder of the presence of the poor is not a statement of apathetic resignation to the status quo. On the contrary, Jesus, the Great Feeder of Multitudes, reminds us that as long as there are poor and hungry people, we are called to generosity and openhandedness.

A MIRACULOUS NEW VISION EMERGES

Faith-based advocacy for foreign nutrition assistance and domestic food programs is yielding results in the battle against stunting, malnutrition, and infant mortality. A prophetic focus on hunger positively affects all facets of society, from maternal health and educational achievement to the efficacy of treatments for HIV/AIDS and other infectious diseases to even the growth of GDP.

Tragically, far too many societies today still have a "hunger season." Food is the first medicine. Malnutrition is a real crisis that can be ended in our day. But just as despair is the enemy of hope, complacency is the enemy of change. We must not relent.

As Christians, we have a moral imperative to advocate for nutrition that sustains all human life. Such advocacy is one of love. It transcends political affiliations and denominational allegiances. It dares to dream of a day where every child and every parent, in every village, city, and town all over the world, has enough to eat every day, where food deserts are extinct and malnutrition is a sad memory, and where no one goes to bed hungry.

When I was a boy making mayonnaise sandwiches, I didn't know someone was speaking up for me. The voices that protected the safety net that, in turn, protected my struggling family changed my life. The voices that speak on behalf of Julia and Hector and millions like them are part of a global love revolution that relentlessly is dreaming an impossible dream and casting a fresh global vision. As Victor Hugo once wrote, "There is one thing stronger than all the armies in the world, and that is an idea whose time has come." They are singing a new song. Can you hear them?

Can you hear the chorus of mothers and fathers, NGOs, religious communities, government officials, businesses, and corporate leaders refusing to let hunger win?

Can you hear their song about the end of hunger as it grows louder, pushing toward the crescendo—the tipping point, after which all the multitudes will be fed?

And I know if I'll only be true, to this glorious quest, that the world will be better for this . . .

Lend your voice to the fight to end global hunger. Join us!

THE BREAD OF HEAVEN

JONATHAN MARTIN

At the center of the Christian faith there is not an idea, a concept, a theology, a doctrine, or a dogma. If you travel through all the ancient texts, sail the rivers of all the great Christian traditions, walk with all the saints throughout the ages, they all lead back to one place: the table of Christ.

The path does not lead to explanations, but to the Eucharist.

The mystery at the very center of the Christian faith is a meal.

You can't comprehend it; you can only taste it.

How is it possible that all the grand existential and theological questions can come down to something as elemental as bread and wine?

All the major religions rightly claim that God—on some level—can be known though nature, reason, and experience. But the claim peculiar to Christianity is that Christ is known through eating and drinking. Jesus is the God whose crumbs get between your teeth and beneath your tongue.

The body of God is offered to satiate our hunger.

I have heard it said that Christians, with regard to Scripture, are "the people of the book." "The book" is vitally important, but it is the table even more so than the text that is the center of the faith, around which all Christian life and practice are oriented. The core of Christian faith is not an idea, but a practice. We are the people of the bread.

•   •   •

If Christian spirituality is less about thinking than about eating and drinking, it makes sense then, that the way Christians respond to hunger takes on heightened significance. The stakes are higher when it's all about bread.

When the Israelites had no food, God provided manna in the wilderness.

The Psalmist said, "I was young and now I am old, yet I have never seen the righteous forsaken or their children begging for bread"—which only meant he had not lived long enough (Psalm 37:25). Because the time will come when the righteous seemingly are forsaken, and God's seed does in fact beg for bread.

Jesus' birthplace of Bethlehem literally means "the house of bread."

When Jesus takes the loaves and the fishes, breaks them, and passes them to the hungry multitude gathered impatiently in front of him, he makes those loaves and fishes into a love feast.

He teaches his disciples to pray, "Give us this day our daily bread."

Not long after that, Jesus breaks the bread with his rough carpenter's hands, and something about his tearing of the bread tears the hearts of the disciples. There is something both tragic and comic about how he offers it to them: "This is my body, which is broken for you."

After the worst thing that could happen already has happened, after they've watched Jesus of Nazareth be crucified, two disciples walk with God on the road to Emmaus . . . but they do not know it. Only later, when they sit around a table, and watch him break the bread, do they finally recognize resurrection: "It's him!"

The bread is broken and offered again, through the trembling hands of an old priest: "The body of Christ, the bread of heaven." Sometimes, a man or woman who eats of the loaf recognizes resurrection too.

Then the end comes, and the humble king—who is love incarnate—calls all created things into account. On what basis will he judge us?

"When I was hungry, did you give me food?"

For those who travel the way of Jesus, bread is not just a sacrament—bread is salvation itself.

• • •

It doesn't matter to God so much what you do with your piety, what you do with your prayers, what you do with your feelings of devotion. The question God asks his people—as they continue to perform their lavish rituals and offer their ceremonial praise—is, "but, what are you going to do with *your bread?*"

Hence the prophetic agenda of the prophet Isaiah:

Is such the fast that I choose,
    a day to humble oneself?
Is it to bow down the head like a bulrush,
    and to lie in sackcloth and ashes?
Will you call this a fast,
    a day acceptable to the LORD?

Is not this the fast that I choose:
    to loose the bonds of injustice,
    to undo the thongs of the yoke,
to let the oppressed go free,
    and to break every yoke?
Is it not to share your bread with the hungry,
    and bring the homeless poor into your house;

when you see the naked, to cover them,
>   and not to hide yourself from your own kin?
> Then your light shall break forth like the dawn,
>   and your healing shall spring up quickly;
> your vindicator shall go before you,
>   the glory of the LORD shall be your rear guard.
> Then you shall call, and the LORD will answer;
>   you shall cry for help, and he will say, Here I am.

> If you remove the yoke from among you,
>   the pointing of the finger, the speaking of evil,
> if you offer your food to the hungry
>   and satisfy the needs of the afflicted,
> then your light shall rise in the darkness
>   and your gloom be like the noonday. (Isaiah 58:5-10 NRSV)

The God who Christians worship does not need anything we have to offer.

Chris E. W. Green summarizes Isaiah's prophetic vision in *Surprised by God:*

> Piety does not please God; only charity does. Whatever good they do for us, and however crucial they are to our witness to others, we do God no favors with our songs, our prayers, our fasts, our offerings, our sermons. He has no need of gifts from us, even if he delights in receiving them when they are offered faithfully. It is for our own good and for the good of others that he calls us to offer our bodies as living sacrifices.[1]

What will you do with your bread?
Did you share it?

The empire controls its subjects through the politics of scarcity. God's economy knows only the politics of abundance. To follow Jesus is to believe there will always be enough. For everyone.

•   •   •

The prayer Christians have prayed for two thousand years says, "Thy kingdom come, thy will be done, on Earth as it is heaven." This is not a passive prayer, waiting on divine action; rather it is a way of re-aligning ourselves with the purposes of God in the world. Christians are called to participate in the reign of God in the world, to cooperate with it—in the words of the apostle Paul, to be colaborers with God.

Therefore, for people of faith, the call to end global hunger is not peripheral or auxiliary. It is fair to say it is a moral and theological imperative, but even that falls short of capturing the fullness that Christian witness entails. Ending hunger is not just something Christian faith demands. It is the very shape of Christian faith itself.

To be a Christian is to live in *imitatio Christi*—to live in imitation of the Christ. We feed the multitudes, because it is what we saw him do. We make space for others at the table of grace, because it is what we saw him do. We offer our own lives to be "blessed, broken, and distributed," to use Henri Nouwen's phrase, because it is what we saw him do.

"If you love me," Jesus said to Simon Peter, "feed my lambs" (John 21:15). He did not say if you love me, "think about me a lot," or "write new worship songs about me," or "make me more famous."

If you love me, Peter, you will act on my behalf. . . . You will feed my sheep.

Though this charge rightly serves as a metaphor for many ways the people of God are to be cared for pastorally, it is noteworthy that the imagery is not abstract, but embodied, material, physical. The call is not exclusively to feed the hungry, the call is certainly not less than that—it is one, if not the only dimension, of Christian worship and discipleship.

●   ●   ●

For people of the bread, it is not surprising that the Christian story ends with a feast, in John's apocalypse—the marriage supper of the Lamb. Whenever Christians gather to break bread and drink wine together, the future feast not only is anticipated, it is also participated in. In the Eucharist, we taste the future, when the table of God will be spread in fullness, and the reign of God will be complete. That table gives us a window into a future in which there is no hunger, so that we might begin to imagine such a future in the world right now.

Whenever we eat and drink at his table, we are charged again to take the bread of life through which we have received God's mercy, and go, in Christ's name, to take his love feast into the present.

In Anglican liturgy for the Eucharist, the priest again says, "The body of Christ, the bread of heaven," and offers the parishioner the consecrated wafer. God also speaks these words over the world, but instead of giving a wafer—he gives the world the church.

If we love him . . . *we will feed his starving sheep.*

PART 2

THE FIRST ONE THOUSAND DAYS: YOUNG WOMEN, MOTHERS, AND CHILDREN

I AM GITA

ROGER THUROW

LUCKNOW, India—**A young mother,** only twenty-two years old, sat on the edge of a hospital bed, her six-week-old daughter swaddled tightly to her chest. Mother and daughter had been inseparable, bound by this skin-to-skin contact since the birth, when the baby weighed just nine hundred grams, or slightly less than two pounds. She constantly needed her mom's warmth and milk.

"I'm Gita," the mother announced to a group of visitors. Her daughter didn't have a name yet—Gita said she wanted to wait until she knew her baby would survive. She was playing a board game, Snakes and Ladders, with another mother who also cradled a low birth weight child. Gita was in high spirits. "I've won three out of four games," she said.

But there was a greater reason for her joy. Her daughter had been weighed again that morning, and the news was encouraging. "She is 1,730 grams now," Gita proclaimed with great pride.

The baby's birth weight had nearly doubled. Another three hundred grams and mom could think about taking her daughter home—and finally giving her a name.

Some of the material in this chapter was adapted from Roger Thurow, *The First 1,000 Days: A Crucial Time for Mothers and Children—and the World* (New York: PublicAffairs, 2016).

In India's maternity wards, the scales tell the story of the country's—and the world's—battle against malnutrition. Malnutrition remains a leading cause globally of nearly half of all deaths of children under the age of five.

In India, more than one-fifth of all babies come into the world with a low birth weight (less than five-and-a-half pounds by international standards). As infants, 21 percent suffer from wasting, or severe underweight according to height. By the time they reach five years of age, nearly 40 percent are stunted either physically, cognitively, or both.

Much of this is due to diets lacking the vital vitamins and nutrients that fuel healthy and strong growth and development. India is home to more than one-third of the world's malnourished children, and a quarter of the world's newborn deaths.

Anemia plagues more than half of Indian women of reproductive age, and nearly 60 percent of all children under age five. Nearly one-quarter of women have a low body mass index. Aggravating the malnutrition are widespread poor sanitation and hygiene, which lead to parasites and water-borne diseases that rob a person's body of whatever nutrients they may consume.

Gita, who comes from an impoverished rural area in the state of Uttar Pradesh, was malnourished and anemic when she was pregnant, and she gave birth a month prematurely. She and her daughter were rushed to the capital city of Lucknow and its District Women's Hospital. A large sign hanging in the hallway of its maternity ward heralds a new treatment the hospital is pioneering: "KMC Unit," shorthand for Kangaroo Mother Care, so named because swaddled newborns resemble joeys (baby kangaroos) in their mothers' pouches. Such skin-to-skin swaddling immediately after birth is more conducive for breastfeeding, helping to encourage weight gain and to prevent hypothermia.

While they nurse their babies under the watchful eye of a team of nurses and doctors, at the District Women's Hospital new mothers eat a steady diet of nutritious vegetables and fruits—bananas, apples, mangos, whatever is in season—so they can gain strength and also pass the nutrients on to their babies through their breast milk. Even though India is the world's second largest producer of fruits and vegetables, many families cannot afford them, creating the paradox of so much malnutrition amid such abundance.

In the past, the odds would have been slim that Gita's baby would survive, but the new mother was encouraged by the statistics she learned from the nurses: 936 severely underweight babies were treated in the KMC ward, and 850 had survived since it opened twenty months earlier in 2016. The KMC treatment is now a centerpiece of the Indian government's National Nutrition Mission, which aims to end the tragic and costly consequences of hunger and malnutrition.

A particular focus of the new nutrition strategy is given to the first one thousand days of life—the time from when a mother first becomes pregnant to the second birthday of her child. This is the most important time for individual human development, when the foundation for good physical growth is laid, when the brain is growing most rapidly and expansively, and when the immune system strengthens for a life of good health. It is the time that determines a child's ability to learn in school, perform at a future job, and ward off chronic disease as an adult.

Good nutrition is essential to fuel all of that growth. Any prolonged bout of malnutrition in the first one thousand days leads to stunting, both physical and cognitive. While the clinical definition of stunting is being too short for one's age, in reality, by the time a child reaches the age of two, stunting usually means a life sentence of underachievement.

Today, globally, one in four children under the age of six is stunted—imagine the lost opportunities—which is why the first one thousand days of a child's life also are the most important for the healthy development of families, communities, nations, and the world as a whole.

● ● ●

In reporting for my book *The First 1,000 Days: A Crucial Time for Mothers and Children—And the World*, I followed moms and their children in India, Uganda, Guatemala, and Chicago on their one-thousand-day journeys.

I expected to find many differences between the mothers and children in the varied locations, but was surprised to discover just as many commonalities, chief among them the hope for every child who comes into the world to achieve all that is possible. It is the most widely shared human aspiration. And when it doesn't happen, we all bear the burden.

A stunted child anywhere in our world becomes a stunted child everywhere. We all share in the cost of lower education, reduced labor productivity, and escalating health care costs. The impact of a stunted child rolls through time and across societies and around the world like the ripples that spread from a single pebble cast into a still pond.

It begins with an individual boy or girl. A child with stunted cognitive development has difficulty learning in school and drops out early, which diminishes the child's prospect for success in the labor force. A study in eastern Guatemala that now spans a half-century has found that children who were well nourished in their first one thousand days completed a couple more grades of school than malnourished children. As adults, the better-nourished group earned 20 to 40 percent more in wages, and were less likely to develop a chronic illness.

Next, the impact spreads to the stunted child's family members, who are likely to earn less than a full wage and incur higher health care costs, in turn making it more difficult for any of them to climb out of poverty.

For many families, the effects of malnutrition and stunting steamroll through the generations in an accumulation of historical insults: stunted girls grow up to be stunted women who give birth to underweight babies who themselves are stunted. And the vicious cycle grinds on.

The ripples from stunting then engulf the community at large, for where there is one malnourished child, there certainly are more. Labor pools are depleted, productivity is sapped, and economic growth lags.

The exponential reach of stunting then continues to radiate outward, crippling entire countries and even continents. Nations with high childhood stunting rates calculate that they annually lose between 5 percent and 16 percent of their gross domestic product to low labor productivity, high health care expenditures, and other effects of malnutrition. Sub-Saharan Africa and South Asia—where aggregate malnutrition stands at about 40 percent and stunting rates are the highest in the world—each lose an estimated 11 percent of their economic activity every year.

Why do some countries and regions of the world remain poor? Because their mothers and children are malnourished and stunted. Because they have a lousy first one thousand days.

Which brings us to stunting's final, devastating ripple effect. According to the World Bank, the cumulative toll of the individual, family, community, and national costs imposes a significant drag on global productivity, international trade, and health care, stunting the world economy by about $3 trillion a year.

While that is a massive number, perhaps the greatest costs of malnutrition and stunting remain immeasurable.

A poem never written.

A song never sung.

A story never told.

A technology never invented.

A building never designed.

A mystery never solved.

A horizon never explored.

An idea never formed.

An inspiration never shared.

An innovation never nurtured.

A cure never discovered.

Imagine what a child might have achieved for all of humankind were she not stunted?

• • •

It's a thought that haunts Dr. Vishwajeet Kumar, an Indian physician who studied and worked in the United States before returning home to tackle the problem of infant mortality in a rural area of the state of Uttar Pradesh.

In Uttar Pradesh, among the poorest regions in India, nearly 55 percent of children younger than three years old were stunted, 42 percent were underweight, and 85 percent suffered from some level of anemia—and those were the children who survived the first months of life.

The newborn mortality rate in the area where Vishwajeet set up his practice was exceedingly high—more than eighty out of every thousand live births. The residents largely believed such infant deaths were fated. But Vishwajeet insisted they were preventable.

Your babies didn't have to die, he told the mothers. *You have the power to ensure they will live.* Vishwajeet's challenge was to move the women and their communities from a state of fatalism to a state of control. To do this, he forged an alliance between modern medicine, community beliefs, and government.

As he began his work, Vishwajeet likened himself to an amateur diver, exploring a new world of strange phenomena. What he discovered in the villages were traditional practices and superstitions, deeply rooted in the region's caste system, culture, and spirituality, that were having a profound impact in the one thousand days. Folk wisdom and common custom encouraged families to make choices discordant with all he had learned in medical school.

More than 80 percent of women still were insisting on delivering their babies at home, even with the proliferation of clinics and hospitals in the countryside. The newborns would be taken from their mothers and thoroughly washed—sometimes heavily scrubbed, even cleansed with mud from a pond—and then left on their own, unclothed, lying on the ground for up to an hour, while the home birth attendants turned to caring for the mothers, as the risk to her life after giving birth was perceived to be higher. This washing and scrubbing was a ritual meant to cleanse away evil spirits, but it dangerously exposed the babies to deadly hypothermia and infection.

Breastfeeding didn't begin for several hours, at the earliest, or in some instances several days; less than 20 percent of newborns in Shivgarh were breastfed immediately. Instead, the first breast milk, containing the antibody-rich colostrum, was discarded because it was considered part of the afterbirth and therefore "unclean." The first liquids a baby received would be cow's milk, water (unpurified, straight from the well), or a drop of honey.

Vishwajeet's team of medical scientists worked with local community leaders to identify a common objective: improve infant survival. Next, they aligned the traditional belief that evil spirits (known as *jamoga*) harm newborns, with the scientific, medical knowledge that infections cause harm to newborns. Infections were *jamoga* too,

Vishwajeet explained, and with this patients began referring to infections as "germ*oga*."

Together, Vishwajeet and community leaders designed a package of behavioral changes—hygienic delivery, light cleansing of the newborn instead of the traditional thorough scrubbing, skin-to-skin contact between mother and child, and immediate breastfeeding with the colostrum—that could conquer the evils (by any name) that contributed to infant deaths.

Vishwajeet named his budding organization the Community Empowerment Lab. But in homes up and down dusty village streets, the women called it, simply, *Saksham* (meaning "empowerment").

When working with the communities, Vishwajeet's favorite visual aid was a mother's own hand with her fingers spread wide. "There are five secrets to success," he would tell the women, assigning one secret to each finger. "One, love. Two, warmth. Three, food—breast milk. Four, hygiene. Five, care—know the signs when your baby is sick and go to the doctor. These behaviors are all in your control. They are in your hands."

It was a revolutionary concept—empowering mothers—in a country where women often have little say in their own homes, even when it comes to reproductive and family planning decisions. And yet, the plan worked.

Within sixteen months, neonatal mortality in the *Saksham* villages was cut in half—forty-one deaths per one thousand live births, compared to eighty-four in neighboring villages where the changes hadn't yet been introduced. Maternal deaths during childbirth became ever rarer. Local government followed *Saksham*'s lead and incorporated the basic tenets of care for pregnant women and their newborn children into the state's public programs, including the Kangaroo Mother Care units.

The Indian government, through its National Nutrition Mission, has set ambitious goals for the next three years: reduce stunting, undernutrition, and low birth weight by six percent; lower the prevalence of anemia among young children and women of child-bearing years by nine percent; and reduce stunting among children under the age of six from the 2016 level of 38.4 percent to 25 percent.

India has made steady progress since 2005, when its stunting rate hovered at nearly 50 percent. But has it come too late for the children on the KMC ward? The odds that they will survive are improving, but will they thrive? Or has stunting already given them a life sentence of underachievement?

The answers to those questions will determine not just India's future, but our own. For a single child to lose a chance at greatness is a loss for all of us.

A THOUSAND DAYS AND A MILLION QUESTIONS

CATHLEEN FALSANI

I **was not present** at my son's birth.

On the day Vasco came into this world, I was at home in the suburbs of Chicago, 8,600 miles away from Blantyre, Malawi, where his first mother, Edina, birthed him at home or perhaps, however unlikely, in a small hospital a few miles away from the clutch of mud-and-wattle huts where she lived with extended family.

I don't know how much Vasco weighed or how long he was at birth. I don't know whether his was an easy labor or a hard one, whether Edina was attended by a midwife or her older sister or a neighbor or one of the Italian nuns from that hospital up the way. I don't know what day, month, or time of the year he was born or even what year it was with any certainty, although I believe it was 1999.

I don't know what Edina ate while she was pregnant, whether she was able to consume enough nutritious foods to keep her healthy and allow the baby growing inside of her to thrive. I don't know if she had access to any vitamins or supplements. I don't know if she ever saw a doctor—before, during, or after she gave birth to Vasco.

I do know my son was born with a ventricular septal defect—a hole in his heart—a congenital defect that is common all over the world (including in Chicago) and that probably had nothing to do with

Edina's own health or nutrition or prenatal care. But it might have. The doctors don't know; no one knows, for sure.

I do know that Edina had given birth at least once before Vasco—she had another son, Juma, who is about two years older than Vasco. Juma's father was a man called Charlie. She had at least two more children after Vasco, but they died in infancy. Two babies. Both girls. That much Vasco remembers. And then Edina died. Vasco's only clear memory of his mother is from her funeral, tied to his grandmother's back with a colorful cloth *chitenge*, watching the mourners weep as the funeral procession made its way by torchlight through his tiny ancestral village.

There are no pictures of Vasco as a newborn, no video of his first steps or his terrible twos. No photographs of him existed at all, in fact, until I took a few snapshots of the beautiful boy with the huge eyes and regal air the day my husband and I met him in Blantyre when he was about seven years old and desperately sick. He was the size of an average three-year-old American kid, even though he was the age of a second grader. He was small—at the time perhaps three feet tall and weighing maybe thirty-five pounds soaking wet—because there had been no medical interventions available to him or his family to help fix or even treat that hole in his heart. I'd later learn that he had the lung capacity of someone with end-stage emphysema and that his heart was so enlarged from years of working so hard, his ribcage bowed outward on his left side. He also had contracted malaria at least twice and somehow survived. Somehow.

Lord, have mercy.

By the time we met, Vasco had been an orphan for some time. Edina had died when he was perhaps two-and-a-half years old, and Vasco's biological father, a man called Sylvester, died a few years after that. I don't know for sure how Edina and Sylvester died, although we suspect it was related to HIV/AIDS, a disease that ravaged an entire generation in Malawi as it did in much of sub-Saharan Africa. Edina's surviving siblings won't say it was AIDS. Instead they claim it was encephalitis, an inflammation of the brain that often is caused by a virus and also is a common side effect of HIV infection, that took their sister's life.

Apparently, Sylvester had another family a few hours south of Blantyre, where Vasco, Juma, and Edina lived. He was a pieceworker and sometimes drove or worked on a truck, meaning that he was on the road a lot. In the 1990s, in many parts of sub-Saharan Africa, HIV and AIDS had spread quickly among truck drivers and traveling workers who frequented prostitutes or were otherwise sexually promiscuous along their journeys. But I don't know if that's what happened to Sylvester. Vasco has memories of his father being strong and lean, with lots of muscles. He worked hard, and Vasco remembers having plenty of food when he lived with Sylvester. One day, his father went away to work in the south and never returned. Months later, Vasco's family in Blantyre heard he had died.

Christ, have mercy.

For extended periods of time, from about the age of five until he was nearly eight years old, Vasco lived alone on the streets of one of the poorest cities in the world, fending for himself, finding food and water and shelter as he could—a tiny, sick, brave, and mighty boy who probably shouldn't have lived long enough to meet his forever parents. But he did.

Thanks be to God.

I didn't become Vasco's mother until he was nine years old. I missed those crucial first one thousand days by at least six years. I won't ever know what his infancy was like—was he colicky? Did he suck his thumb? Was he an easy baby?—what his first word was, how old he was when he learned to walk, or how and when he first was diagnosed with the heart defect.

I won't ever know for sure whether Edina breastfed him, although she probably did as about 95 percent of Malawian mothers do—one of the highest scores for breastfeeding in the developing world. According to a Save the Children report, "Nutrition in the First 1,000 Days," at the age of two, 77 percent of Malawian children still receive some of their nutrition from breast milk.[1] By the time Vasco was two, sadly, Edina likely was sick or dying. I don't know what she fed him when he was weaned and moved on to solids. Was she able to provide him more than the maize paste and greens that are the staples of the Malawian diet? Did he get sufficient protein to help his young brain grow? Cassava? Sweet potatoes? I don't know.

At the time of Vasco's birth in 1999, Malawi had one of the highest infant mortality rates in the world—107 deaths per one thousand live births. Today, that same rate has dropped dramatically to thirty-nine deaths per one thousand live births, and that is a 72 percent reduction from 1990 when the rate was 138 deaths per one thousand live births.[2] In this regard, Malawi is considered a success story by the World Health Organization, UNICEF, and others.

But the country still has one of the highest rates of stunted children in the world—more than half of all Malawian children (54 percent) are stunted, according to a 2015 report on research commissioned by the African Union.[3] Stunting, meaning a child has low height and size for his or her age, is the result of children missing out on vital nutrients when they are in utero through the first two years of their lives—those magical, all-important, first one thousand days.

The effects of stunting, including frequent illness, poor cognitive ability, difficulty in school, and lackluster performance at work, can be devastating and last for a lifetime. That same study, titled "The Cost of Hunger in Africa: The Social and Economic Impact of Child Undernutrition in Malawi," found that nearly 60 percent of adult Malawians still suffered the effects of stunting, which in turn affects the workforce (about two-thirds of the population works in manual labor) and overall productivity. In 2012 alone, Malawi lost more than 10 percent of its gross domestic product (about $600 million) as a result of child undernutrition.[4]

Whatever Edina was able to do for Vasco in those first one thousand days—"the window of opportunity to build healthier and more prosperous futures," as one UNICEF report calls it—as her health was failing and he was struggling to thrive against the complications presented by a significant heart defect, it apparently was enough. Because despite his heart problems (which were fixed beautifully by the miracle of open-heart surgery when he came to Chicago in late April 2009), Vasco has grown into a strong, athletic, healthy, bright, extremely fit young man who learns things quickly, thinks deeply, and has seemingly infinite reserves of patience, grace, and peace.

When he arrived in Chicago, he was nine years old, weighed forty-two pounds, and was about forty inches tall. He couldn't read or write in any language and he had attended school only sporadically over the years in Blantyre because of his health and homelessness. Those first few weeks, before his heart surgery, I carried him on my hip like a toddler when he was too tired to walk, which was often. In the first six months after his surgery, with the help of a working heart and a hearty, healthy, balanced diet, Vasco grew six inches. He blossomed through a new shoe size about every six weeks, and my husband still jokes that if you listened carefully at night, you could hear his feet growing.

Three months after his arrival in the United States, in September 2009, he enrolled as a fourth grader in our local public school. By Christmas he was reading on his own and had learned to swim and surf, and his American Youth Soccer Organization (AYSO) soccer team, the Fat Pandas, had won the town championship.

Today, Vasco is five-foot-nine-and-a-half, trim and muscular. He's quick-witted and kind, curious and reasonably studious. And while math and science are not his strong suits (they're not mine, either), he holds his own in the humanities and the arts. He will tell you his favorite high school subject was history and that he is interested in studying psychology in college. In June 2018, he graduated from high school and decided to take a gap year to explore his options before enrolling at a four-year school. He intends to return to Malawi someday sooner rather than later to help make life better for children whose first one thousand days should be filled with hope and potential, not insecurity and unanswerable questions.

Vasco is the miraculous exception to the rule. He shouldn't have to be.

And with God's grace, soon he won't be.

NAME: Vasco
AGE: 19
LOCATION: Blantyre, Malawi

What's the longest you've ever gone without eating? Two hours? A day?

Have you ever gone a week without eating? I bet not.

In my younger years when I lived in Malawi, Africa, I did not grow up in a wealthy family. After my birth parents died, I lived with my uncle and brother and a few other more distant relatives where I was the second youngest in the group.

I had to walk miles to get to the nearest market. As a growing kid, I needed to eat a lot of food to keep my energy up. Sadly, that was not the way life was for me. Most days, I would eat maybe a packet of biscuits (flat, brown cookies) or two, and that would be all for the rest of the day.

Sometimes I would have to rely on that packet of biscuits for the next day as well.

In fact, what I remember most about growing up in Blantyre, Malawi, is that I was hungry every day. But I never complained or whined. Instead, I tried my best to stay positive and pray that God would provide me with some strength to get through the week or just the next day.

I went to the market almost every day to find some sort of scraps or leftovers and sometimes I would ask people for money. This went on for the first eight years of my life. My uncle would feed me sometimes, but I was never a priority. To him, I was just a kid that got handed down because I had nowhere else to go.

The days that I never had anything to eat at all were the hardest. My stomach would hurt a lot, and it was a pain that would last most of the day. The very worst of those days was when I would see other people eating food when I had nothing. I would watch them and wish that were me.

When I reached the age of nine, I was very skinny. I weighed less than forty pounds and I was less than four feet tall. What I remember most was being smaller than other kids. I was like a feather.

In 2009, I came to the United States for heart surgery and was adopted. Eating daily—multiple times a day—was a weird transition for me. It was strange because I went from eating just a tiny amount or nothing at all for weeks on end to eating in the morning, in the afternoon, and at night. Here, there is always food. I began to realize how privileged and blessed I was. Many times, after dinner, I would think back to the days when I would walk for miles and hope to find something, anything, that would last me just for that day.

A couple of years after I became an American, our youth group at church had a fast that lasted twenty-four hours to raise awareness about global hunger. During our fast, we made food for the homeless people in our town, but we were not allowed to eat anything—we could only drink water. I recall how I hated fasting that day. We were making food that we weren't allowed to eat. What the heck? The smell of the food made it so much worse. I realized I was angry because I had become used to eating every day.

In the United States, we are used to a life where food is easy to get and we forget that there are a lot of kids who are starving and trying to find literal scraps to make ends meet. I know what it's like to go hungry for days and even weeks.

My message is simple: *please* don't waste food or throw away something that has been in your fridge for one day. Think of the kids who are starving and would love to eat what's perfectly good. And at the very least, for those reading my story, please take the time to pray for those kids who aren't as privileged as you.

TO END PREVENTABLE DEATHS IN MOTHERS AND CHILDREN, WE MUST END HUNGER AND MALNUTRITION

MARK K. SHRIVER

Oumar's life was on the line.

His mother, Mariama, rushed him to a Save the Children–supported hospital in rural Niger after growing increasingly concerned for her baby boy. A terrible drought had destroyed their crops, leaving them with almost nothing to eat. Then Oumar became dangerously ill from drinking dirty water. He was wasting away to skin and bones, suffering from acute malnutrition.

"He started being sick with vomiting and diarrhea," Mariama said. "Before he got sick, he was a normal weight—not too fat, not too skinny, but just right. Oumar was sick all the time, and it broke my heart. I was always worried about him and was afraid that he might not make it."

Oumar received medicine to treat his fever and stomach infection. Then his appetite came back, and he enjoyed eating a specially formulated peanut paste called Plumpy Nut, designed to give him all the nutrients he needed. Now on the road to recovery at age two, Oumar can focus again on being a kid.

"Oumar's personality is joyful. He's usually very friendly and smiling. He visits his friends and playmates crawling around like a little chief," Mariama said. "Oumar likes to play with the older kids. He loves making sand castles using cans and knickknacks he finds around the village."

Not every child with severe acute malnutrition is so fortunate. Millions of families around the world face the tragedy of losing a child unnecessarily every year. Malnutrition is the underlying cause of 45 percent of deaths in children younger than the age of five—a statistic we easily can reduce.

Every day, fifteen thousand children throughout the world die from easily treatable illnesses such as pneumonia, malaria, and malnutrition. And eight hundred mothers die every day from complications related to pregnancy and childbirth. This is tragic, but fortunately, because of US leadership, we have made great progress in saving the lives of children and mothers around the world. Since 1990, we have reduced the number of preventable child deaths by half and maternal deaths by 40 percent.

In 2015, world leaders, including the United States, signed onto the Sustainable Development Goals that promised to end poverty, hunger, all forms of malnutrition, and preventable child and maternal deaths. Tackling malnutrition is key in reaching these goals.

POVERTY AND MALNUTRITION ARE INTERLINKED

Children's health and development depend on their mothers' health, before and during pregnancy. A mother who is chronically malnourished is more likely to give birth to an underweight baby. An underweight baby is less likely to grow and develop physically and cognitively, and is more susceptible to chronic malnutrition, illness, and death.

Poverty is a primary driver of hunger. Countries and regions that experience high levels of poverty tend to see more mothers and children living with hunger and malnutrition. With a very low income, it is hard for a family to feed itself, let alone buy good, nutritious foods.

Malnourished children struggle more in school and tend to get jobs that do not pay as well as those of their well-nourished peers. Later in life, they cannot support or feed their families, creating another malnourished and impoverished generation. Nutrition for mothers and children means a future of greater opportunity and well-being for all.

ENDING MALNUTRITION IS KEY
TO ENDING PREVENTABLE DEATHS

The first one thousand days of a child's life—between pregnancy and a child's second birthday—are the "window of opportunity" to ensure healthy growth and development of a child. During this period, it is crucial for mothers and their young children to have access to good nutrition. Poor nutrition for both a mother and child during this window is associated with slowed physical and cognitive development, a phenomenon known as stunting.

A common result of chronic malnutrition, stunting affected 155 million children younger than age five in 2016. Stunted children face additional hardships such as difficulty in school, lowered productivity and work performance, and loss of wages in adulthood. When children receive poor nutrition during the first one thousand days of their lives, it also affects the development of strong immune systems, making children more likely to contract diseases, and perpetuating a cycle of poor health issues that is difficult to break. Health and nutrition interventions for young mothers must be implemented during these one thousand days.

ROLE OF THE UNITED STATES GOVERNMENT IN INCREASING THE VISIBILITY OF MALNUTRITION

The United States is a signatory on global commitments to end poverty, hunger, and all forms of malnutrition, and preventable child and maternal deaths. We have been a strong leader in the fight against global hunger and malnutrition, in promoting optimal maternal and child health.

The global food crisis in 2008 resulted in renewed attention to food insecurity. This ultimately led to a commitment by President Barack Obama at the G8 Summit in 2009 in L'Aquila, Italy, where the US government pledged to leverage and align substantial funding for a common approach to end hunger and malnutrition. At this meeting, the United States launched a major food security initiative called Feed the Future, which is aimed at combating hunger—including malnutrition—and poverty around the world.

This was followed by the launch of the 1,000 Days Partnership by the governments of the United States and Ireland that, for the first time, raised awareness on the critical need to address malnutrition in mothers and infants during the one-thousand-day period. This initiative also emphasized that nutrition was not just a food issue, but also a health issue.

In 2012, the United States, along with the governments of India and Ethiopia, cohosted the Child Survival Call to Action—a meeting that launched the vision to end preventable child and maternal deaths. For the first time, nutrition-specific interventions were included on the list of key interventions to be scaled up in order to bend the curve on maternal and child deaths. The same year, the United States also committed to six globally agreed upon nutrition targets: a reduction in stunting among children younger than age five, a reduction in incidents of anemia among women of childbearing age, a reduction in low birth weight, no increase in child obesity, an increase in the rate of exclusive breastfeeding for the first six months of life, and a reduction in childhood wasting.

This is terrific progress, but we have much more work to do.

• • •

Joynab, a mother in Bangladesh, does not know about prenatal care because it is not practiced in her community. She received no immunizations or nutritional supplements during her pregnancies. None of her children has been fully vaccinated or received vitamin A supplementation. Her eight-month-old son, Ashim, suffers from frequent fever, diarrhea, and severe acute malnutrition.

US leadership is critical in ensuring Joynab and mothers like her receive good nutrition, and that children such as Oumar and Ashim survive and thrive beyond their fifth birthdays. The United States must continue to be a global leader in this space and fulfill its commitments to end preventable child and maternal deaths and all forms of malnutrition.

US partnerships through Feed the Future in countries such as Kenya, Ethiopia, and Bangladesh have resulted in the significant reduction of chronic malnutrition and stunting. For example, between 2011 and 2014, Bangladesh reduced the prevalence of stunting among children by 12 percent. Ethiopia reduced child malnutrition from 44 percent in 2011 to 38 percent in 2016. This means that many more children benefit from the good nutrition, health care, and education that ensure optimal growth and development for their futures.

These are significant reductions in a short amount of time, with a relatively small amount of funding. The US government provides just $125 million annually for nutrition in global health, and $1 billion annually for the entire Feed the Future program, which includes initiatives broader than nutrition. Since 2009, Feed the Future has reached more than eighteen million children.

US foreign assistance programs, particularly maternal and child survival and nutrition, are improving the lives of mothers and children worldwide. These programs have played a significant role in ensuring that children live beyond age five, and that mothers and children grow, develop, and thrive. In all, since 2008, the US Agency for International Development's (USAID) maternal and child survival efforts have saved the lives of more than five million children and two hundred thousand women.

BUILDING SUPPORT IN CONGRESS

Two years ago, Congress passed the Global Food Security Act. This bill calls for a comprehensive, strategic US government approach to reducing global poverty and hunger, achieving food security, fostering agricultural growth, and improving nutritional outcomes—especially for women and children. This was a major victory toward breaking the intergenerational cycles of poverty for the millions of children affected by hunger and malnutrition worldwide.

Congress should build on that critical progress and pass new legislation called the Reach Every Mother and Child Act (Reach Act), which has been introduced in the US Senate and House of Representatives. If passed, the Reach Act would ensure that the United States fulfills its promise to end preventable child and maternal deaths, and improve nutrition by scaling up our successful programs and increasing access to simple, affordable solutions that we know save lives, such as trained community health workers, basic medication, and medical equipment.

Leveraging innovative financing tools to reduce the global financing gap in addressing maternal, newborn, and child health, the Reach Act also would ensure the United States continues to promote a comprehensive, evidence-based approach, where key interventions such as nutrition are prioritized, to ensure that every child survives and thrives.

The bill has significant bipartisan support in both chambers of Congress. It would require the United States to develop a strategy for realizing the bold vision of saving fifteen million children's lives and six hundred thousand women's lives globally. The Reach Act would allow the United States to expand its moral leadership and achieve the national security and economic goals we need to keep us secure.

We all must do our part to ensure mothers and children everywhere have a strong start in life.

AMAZZI

When You Have Enough

E ditors' note: *In 2004, on a trip to Uganda with a delegation from Compassion International, Steve and Debbie Taylor met a little girl named Sarah. At the time, the couple had been married almost twenty years. They had no biological children. They were not looking necessarily to adopt a child either, although the idea did appeal to them.*

Nevertheless, on that visit to Uganda, Sarah, who was perhaps five years old at the time—the youngest and smallest child living at an orphanage near Kampala—made their decision for them. She became Debbie's shadow, following the woman who soon would become her mother around for four hours. Amazzi (the Lugandan language's word for "water") was the first word Sarah spoke to Debbie, as she held up a bright orange plastic cup. A few days later in Kenya, before returning home to Nashville, Debbie asked Steve what he thought about trying to adopt Sarah. Surprised and delighted, he agreed to find out what was possible when they got home. It took some doing (it was difficult to adopt from Uganda and other east African nations at the time because of an absence of clear international adoption laws on the books), but the following year, Debbie and Steve returned to Uganda to adopt Sarah.

The details of those earliest days together are familiar to any family that has adopted an older child internationally, and a common theme of those first experiences—which become family lore—was that they often involved food. Food, despite being left out of Gary Chapman's The Five Love Languages, *most assuredly is one of the most universal ways we communicate love, care, and compassion in any tongue.*

In the early summer of 2018, not long after Sarah had returned home from her first year at college, the Taylors sat down for a group conversation about their experiences with food—and hunger—in Africa and at home in Tennessee.

•   •   •

STEVE: When we finally got approval to proceed with the adoption, we were able to go back to Uganda. Meanwhile, Sarah had no idea that any of this was going on until a friend of ours, an American missionary who had been helping us and was the assistant to the Anglican archbishop of Uganda, went to meet with the house mother at the orphanage, who, of course, knew what was going on. The house mother called Sarah into the office from the playground and said, in Luganda, which was Sarah's native language, "Sarah, would you like to go on an airplane?" And Sarah said, "Yes." Then she said, "Would you like to go to America?" And Sarah said, "Yes." And then she said, "Would you like to live with *muzungus* [the local word for white people]?" Sarah hesitated for a moment, and then replied, "Yes."

So the house mother said, "Okay, you can go back out and play." And Sarah returned to the playground. Then our friend Jennifer turned to the woman and said, "I'm sorry, but there's no way that little girl understands anything you just told her."

But just a few moments later, all the kids from the orphanage started pounding on the windows of the office, shouting: "We want to go to America! We want to go to America!"

Apparently, when Sarah got back to the playground, she said, "Guess where I'm going?" And the kids weren't particularly helpful. They told her that when you go to America, you'll get chicken every day, and you'll get cookies every day, and they give you a car!

SARAH: Yeah. The first two were true. But I'm still saving money for the car.

STEVE: So that's the story of how we became a family. It was 2005.

SARAH: I don't remember that. I can only remember certain things. So, to me, it's just like I've always been in America, even though I know in my head that I haven't.

STEVE: Sarah had a friend she grew up with contact her a few months ago on Facebook.

SARAH: Yeah, he was like my brother when we were at the orphanage. He's one of the only memories I still have from my time in Uganda. I don't remember a lot, but I know he was like my brother, and I lived with him and his grandma before I went to the orphanage with him. He contacted me, and he said, "Sarah, it's me, Joshua. I've been looking for you for so long." We had the same grandma, so he is, I guess, my cousin. Since then, I often get new friend requests from someone in Uganda who had been in the orphanage with me. And they all tell me stories about things that I did.

STEVE: Tell them what Joshua told you about your age.

SARAH: Oh yeah! I was talking to him, and he asked, "How old are you?" And I say, "I turn twenty-one in August." And he says, "No, you can't be twenty-one, because I'm twenty-one, and you were younger than me. You were the youngest kid at the orphanage." I thought, *oh well.* Supposedly, he doesn't know what his birthday is either, but he's sure he's older than me.

I've always thought I was younger, so this doesn't really change anything, because I've always kind of known in my head, you know? But it was good to have it validated.

STEVE: She has a birth certificate, but we were told that in her village those aren't necessarily trustworthy documents. In retrospect, she looked so much younger than seven when we met her. She looked more like five. When we returned to Uganda, she already had lost her front teeth, which, for most kids, happens between five and seven. But we thought (and were told) she was eight. . . . She was really tiny, and we don't know if that might have been because of a nutritional issue.

SARAH: But I didn't look malnourished.

STEVE: No, you didn't look malnourished.

SARAH: I was just really small.

STEVE: Right. Her doctors here in America have never said anything about stunted growth, but it's a good question. I think you were adequately fed at the orphanage.

SARAH: Yeah, I didn't starve.

STEVE: Even when she was younger, before the orphanage, she was taken into a Compassion International day school project, and they would feed her a nutritional meal each day.

SARAH: It's interesting because when I talked to my friend or cousin or whatever he is, Joshua, who was in the orphanage with me, he said, "My sister, I'm so glad I found you. I'm glad that you don't starve like we used to as children." So, I feel like maybe I used to starve, but I myself do not remember that.

STEVE: The first thing, the first word you ever said to Debbie was—what was the word for water?

DEBBIE: *Amazzi*. It was the first time we visited and met Sarah. She wanted to get a drink of water but didn't want to miss out on any of the fun, so she pulled out a plastic cup, and we got a little drink of water from the storage room, and she wiped her lips, and we went back out to the group.

STEVE: So, there was a connection, initially, with water. And then, when we came back to the States—Debbie is a really good cook— there were a lot of food-related connections.

SARAH: I'm just a basic eater. Chicken, rice, meat.

STEVE: Meat was the jackpot—it was a big deal to have meat.

SARAH: But no pork.

STEVE: Yes, and *no pig*. I remember after our first court hearing where we got provisional permission to adopt her, we went out to celebrate at an American-style restaurant in Kampala for breakfast, and I ordered bacon and eggs. Sarah scrutinized my plate, and I said, "Would you like some bacon?" And she nodded her head, so I gave her a piece. As soon as she put it in her mouth, she spit it out and said, "Is pig?" And I said, "Yeah." And she leaned over and said, "Don't eat pig. Is going to sick." Then after she spit it out, she wiped her tongue and her mouth out. So pig was a no-go.

SARAH: And didn't you end up getting sick?

STEVE: Yes, and evidently that was the cause. We later took her to have her first hamburger while we were still in Kampala, and she loved it. The next day she wanted to go back and get another hamburger, but she was still learning basic English and couldn't recall the word. She knew the phrase, "I want," and she knew some other basic nouns, so she put together this sentence: "I want cow on bread." And we got her another hamburger as a reward.

DEBBIE: I have two things in particular that I remember about Sarah when it comes to food: First, she said that when she was living at the orphanage her father would sometimes bring her donuts. (Her biological father died sometime after she was placed in the orphanage when she was maybe four or five years old.) So, for Sarah's first Father's Day in America, we went to Krispy Kreme and got donuts in honor of her dad.

Another incident happened with one of her American babysitters: Sarah wanted an egg, so she cooked her an egg, and Sarah said she was still hungry, so she cooked her another egg. The babysitter ended up making her eight eggs. Sarah was just so pure when it came to things Americans take for granted. She'd never been to McDonald's or had junk food. When she was first introduced to pizza, she devoured an entire pie. This was starting to become her habit, so when I finally told her doctor, he said, "Don't give her the whole pizza. Just give her two or three slices at the most." During the initial months we spent with Sarah in Uganda, she would eat anything and everything we put in front of her.

She and her friend Lydia would sneak in and steal cookies in the afternoon, which, of course, doesn't surprise me at all. She would just power through anything we gave her. And then, once we got to America, she knew what she liked, and I think after all the excitement of having all these different things, she just kind of settled back into what she'd grown up with, which is kind of a bland diet, really. She likes roasted meat and rice, and she *really* likes pizza.

STEVE: We became much more aware of food insecurity during our time in Uganda. What would it be like to grow up not knowing when or even if you'll have another meal? Sarah almost had to be taught that she could trust us to—

DEBBIE: Feed her again.

STEVE: Yes.

•　　•　　•

SARAH: All throughout high school, when I would have to give a speech, I always talked about hunger. Because during that time, I looked up the statistics, and it's crazy. I did one report on hunger and then I looked up how much food Americans waste, and it was a crazy high number. We could feed so many people with the food we waste. But then it's sad too. I realized that I am also one of those statistics. I went from being a statistic in poverty and not having enough to eat, to being a statistic of another kind as an American who *does* waste food all the time without thinking. So, that's kind of crazy, but I definitely think it's an important topic that a lot of people don't know about. . . .

You can give someone in Africa a goat and you can go on a mission trip and take cute photos and give them money, but once you leave they're still going to be poor. They will still go to bed hungry. I think our problem is that we focus more on how mission trips are going to help them and are like a little break for people living in poverty, but in reality, I don't think it really does much. It probably does a lot for the people who are going on the mission trip, and it probably makes for a great college essay. But that kid in Africa is going to remember you for maybe a month, and then he or she will think about why you aren't coming back to visit, and they're still poor and hungry. Instead of going on these trips, I think we need to figure out some way we can all work together with people in poverty, to help them help themselves, you know what I mean? Instead of giving the man a fish . . .

It would be so much better if we worked alongside them and figured out a better way for families to sustain themselves over a lifetime.

DEBBIE: She's always had a tender heart for people who are in need.

SARAH: I love people, and seeing people who are suffering really gets to me. I would have thought I'd need to return to a Third World country to help suffering people, but I can help them in my own downtown. I've always been like that, and I want to go everywhere. India, Sudan, Chicago. Everywhere. I don't think I can change the world by myself, but I can help.

NAME: Nighty
AGE: 35
LOCATION: Pajimo, Uganda

Nighty lives with her five children in a small village called Pajimo, in the Akwang Subcounty of Kitgum district, northern Uganda. Her studies ended in the third year of secondary school when she lost her dad. She had to drop out of school due to lack of money for school fees, and soon eloped with a man. Her first husband lived with her for about four years until he died (about five years ago) from a random gunshot near an army barrack close to her home, leaving her with three kids.

She later got married to a man who gave her two additional children. This new husband has since abandoned her and now lives in town with another woman. Nighty is left to take care of all five kids and to provide for their schooling, meals, and health care.

Nighty yearly struggles to do farming on her own, and occasionally she has to let her two elder daughters cut school in order to help her with the farm work. Nighty's aspiration is to get some oxen to support her open land so that she can live better.

Would you please tell me about a time in your life when you experienced hunger or had food insecurity for yourself or your children?

Nighty: Yes, I've had hunger. In my adulthood and now as a mother. You know, I could have forgotten certain things from when I was a child.

But about hunger, it happened to me, and I am the one who can tell this story better. It was a serious situation in 2017. One day I had nothing to cook for my kids during that hunger period. I decided to go and do casual day labor so that I could get a payment of about 3000 UGX [0.7 USD] to buy food. The price of food in the market was very high. I found that there was nothing to buy. The few cassava that came into the market were raided immediately. People who had money bought it all. That day, I had to return home without anything, and that night my children and I slept hungry. The whole week there was nothing to eat at home. I decided to go and pick any leaf that could be cooked and eaten from the bush. I could boil these leaves and give them to my children so that they could survive. Sometimes I could see them vomit the meals with cassava they ate but I kept on like that because I knew it would help them survive.

I then thought that it may be better for us to move to my mum's village. I decided that I had to move with my kids to my mum's place so that maybe they would help me provide for my kids during this hunger period, but when I reached my mum's place, I found the situation was the same. People could go daily to do casual labor for food, but it was not enough. We were forced to return home. My kids became very weak, and I thought to myself, *what should I do? My kids are going to die.* If it were possible, I would have swallowed them all to keep them as one person. *Or should I kill them and myself so that it all ends here?* I had a lot of thoughts, and as a mother I was totally heartbroken and disgruntled. I was thinking each moment about how I would manage to keep my children alive. I was confused and did not know what to do. I cried and could not cry any more.

When we came back, I had to continue picking leaves and boiling them for my kids. I picked Labakare leaves, wild plants that I was told are edible. This time I boiled them plain without salt because I also did not have any money to buy salt. My kids had to take them and went to sleep without bread/posho.

How many days did you take at your mum's place with the kids because of the problems of hunger?

Nighty: We had to return the following day. I thought it was better for the kids to die in their own home or their dad's place. We returned from that place, called Oryang Ogom, a village eight kilometers from here.

I connected with a friend who allowed me to work for her that day and who then gave me some cassava to cook. The following day I boiled the cassava and gave it to my kids. Due to our prolonged days of hunger, everybody vomited and felt dizzy or lightheaded after eating the cassava. It was so serious that I thought we were all going to die. It's a story that I won't forget.

How many kids did you have at that time?

Nighty: I had five children. I experienced another serious challenge with hunger after delivering my last born in August 2016. I didn't have any capacity to get anything to eat, and yet I had just delivered. You know how a *min-Lanyuru* (mother who has just delivered) wants food. Think about when it's not there. I think this hunger has affected me until now—I have remained weak.

Where was the father of your children?

Nighty: He was around for a few years when we had the first two kids. That was the time I felt supported as he was with me. When I delivered the other two kids, he abandoned me and left for town to live with another woman. He has abandoned me now for the last five years.

He rarely comes to visit, sometimes just once a year. But now, it has been almost two years since he has shown up. So I am the one struggling with the kids. When it's sickness, when it's a lack of food . . . it's on me to shoulder the responsibility. Like for this month (August 2018), three of my kids were admitted to the Health Centre with malaria. He did not come to see them or give us any support. The medical staff attempted to call him, but he did not show up. Sometimes the school administration has sent my kids away for lack of school fees, and they have to stay home until I find the money for their fees. I always struggle and eventually send them back to school each time.

What would you tell Christians in the United States if you had the chance? What would you want them to know about people in other parts of the world who are struggling with hunger?

Nighty: If there is anything they can do, it is good. If there are some people who can help support the education of the children, it is good. If they can give us some food during a hunger period, it is also good, or to start up income-generating activities for women in similar situations. Because the same money you could have used for buying food, you use for paying school fees. Feeding then becomes a problem. You may use the money for buying food. When you have been given food also it can support what you cultivate yourself so that you don't run short of food to eat.

HUNGER AND
SEX TRAFFICKING

NIKOLE LIM

I was in Nairobi, Kenya, bent over buckets of soapy water, scrubbing remnants of dirt out of my pants. Three years ago, I started an organization with the audacious mission of ending the cycle of sexual violence through education and leadership. I had just come back from a home visit with one of the high school girls in my organization who lives in the slums. She was one of our first scholarship recipients. Her name was Jane.

During this home visit, she finally opened up and shared her story with me. I'd known her for three years. Hearing her story for the first time, I was broken. Breathing hard, hands aching, fighting back tears—the task of scrubbing my dirty clothes forced me to identify with a pain I never before had experienced. Hand washing laundry is one of the many things I never have had to do on a regular basis—but it isn't the only thing.

When we met, Jane was just eighteen years old—quiet and shy. A mound of insecurities created a barrier between her and me. Our different upbringings created the crazy intersection separating us, and it was hard to cross.

Our conversation was at a standstill, and we both were stuck at a crossroads. At twenty-two, I hardly knew anything about the oppression that surrounded young women in Kenya. I tried to ask Jane questions about her dreams, but she would answer only with a yes, a no, and perhaps the hint of a hidden smile. I sensed that not only was she fighting against something internal, but she also was battling external factors compounded by a tangled web of other issues my mind could never comprehend—issues that commonly taunt young women living in Nairobi's slums.

I recall when Jane first took me to her home close to Kibera, a slum in Kenya's capital. With more than one million people living there, it was the largest slum in all of eastern Africa. On our way to her home, we passed a butcher, a small shop owner, and a seamstress. We ducked under dripping laundry left drying on a line and jumped across inlets of open sewage. Here, constructed on a foundation of dirt, behind rusty tin sheaths and faded sheets made into curtains, was the house that Jane had lived in since she was two years old.

The entire house was a single room—smaller than my bedroom back at home in the United States.

Two beds, a couch, a chair, a coffee table, a jerry can of water, and a television were placed strategically like Tetris pieces, and a floral bedsheet hung loosely from wall to wall, separating the single room into two even smaller spaces.

"I stay here with my mother and brother," Jane said.

Her mother, who suffered from chronic back pain (the result of hard labor), was out for the day to sell chai (tea) and chapati (fried tortillas) by the side of the road. Her brother also was out looking for manual labor jobs.

Security was low, and the stakes were high—too many times had her family gone without eating to afford the $30 monthly rent. They would burn sugar in a teaspoon and stir it in hot water for flavor because they couldn't afford tea leaves; eat cabbage with nothing because they couldn't afford salt; and boil and eat the remnants of bitter herbs that grew wildly around the edges of the slums if they couldn't afford cabbage.

"To be honest, I lost all hope," Jane said, her face lit by the glow of a single, naked bulb that dangled by a thin cord from the ceiling.

It wasn't an interrogation room, but it felt like it. Jane challenged me with her story. She told me that she was fighting—fighting against pressures no teenager ever should face. She told me about lacking access to clean, running water, which forced her instead to use a public toilet, where she feared being raped. She told me tales of her young friends who sell sex for as little as ten, twenty, maybe fifty cents. She told me about the rampant prostitution in the slums—how school-girls as young as six sell their small bodies for a packet of rice for their family of four.

"What is it like living in the slums?" I asked.

"It's hard, you know, people here—especially girls—they do things like sell their bodies just to get something to eat. It's the only way they can feed their families," Jane answered.

"Have they pressured you?" I said.

"Yeah, all the time, but I can never do that," she said. "I would rather die."

Jane looked down at her thighs tightly pressed together. Her feet bounced up and down. Her eyes darted around the room restlessly, as if she were trying to divert my attention away from her and into the realities of the world outside those tin walls. She was lying to protect me from the truth of her survival.

"How else do you survive?" I asked.

She chuckled and rolled her eyes at my naiveté.

"I wash laundry for people, clean people's houses—you know, the normal things," she said. "I sell vegetables with my mum."

Then she abruptly sighed, and that was my cue to end the invasive questioning.

I was caught asking this vulnerable teenager questions, but, really, I was interrogating myself about the realities of security for young women living in the slums—the accessibility of health care, corrupt police forces, and equal opportunities for and access to a solid education, self-worth, and dignity.

What would I do if I had to choose between using my savings for school tuition fees or a meal for my hungry family?

All of these questions and issues I never had to consider when I was eighteen years old.

Jane and I talked about her dreams and her aspirations, all of which seemingly were out of reach. Her life was infused with challenges and obstacles, fear and loss. She dreamed of working behind the scenes for the news media to expose the truth of how slum life oppresses, assaults, and victimizes women.

But Jane didn't spend time daydreaming. She was too busy trying to navigate her way through a crossroads, caught between her own dreams, however daunting and unattainable they might seem, and her family's dire, daily needs. She put her own dreams behind her in order to fight for her family's survival.

Inspired by her tenacity, my colleagues and I brought Jane into our programs. And she flourished, graduating from high school later that same year. Soon, she enrolled at a university in Nairobi that is well-known for its mass communications program.

A few months after she began her university studies, I returned to her neighborhood to check on Jane and her family. Her brother had tragically died from HIV/AIDS, which left his daughter for Jane to care for.

Jane arrived, huffing and puffing, having hustled on foot to our meeting from her niece's school some distance away. She was radiant and looked amazing, smiling freely and not trying to hide her new-found confidence. She had been to her niece's school to plead with the principal to let her remain in classes for that week, even though her niece's school fees were in arrears. Jane was determined to pay her niece's school balance in full—just $50.

"So, this weekend, I'll try to find some small jobs in the community to do," Jane said, explaining her plan for raising the money. "I usually wash clothes for people in the richer parts of town. I never want to make money the way I was forced to do when I was in high school."

Hidden behind her unfettered smile was a story I had never heard, one she had tried to forget and had hidden from me before. Her new-found calling was asking her to speak her truth: when she was fourteen, Jane met a boy. Actually, he was more man than boy, much older than she was, and he would often take her to Nairobi's night-clubs to escape the pressures of slum life—pressures that taunted, mocked, and tormented her, doubts and deceptions that wanted her to believe her dreams and ideals were impossibilities. Escape seemed necessary, and Jane trusted the young man.

Until one night, he raped her, initiating her into the way of life she most feared.

He attempted to shatter her sense of worth even as he tried to squash her hopes and dreams, whispering lies, trying to get her to believe the only way she could continue her education was to work the streets to pay for her school fees.

Once again, Jane found herself at a crossroads, unable to make a way forward, and yet she resisted. Weeks later, she found she was pregnant, and, succumbing to pressure from friends and hoping to temper the pain of lost dreams, she had an abortion.

She prayed she could continue on in hiding, but then Jane became extremely ill with intense stomach pains and violent vomiting. She returned to the clinic only to learn that she had been carrying twins and, though one had been aborted successfully, the other, while dead, was still stuck in her womb.

Feeling as if she had reached the point of no return, Jane gave up hope and gave in to despair. After all, she thought, most of her friends felt like they had no other option but to live like this, as if her dreams were dead, stillborn.

Stuck. Coerced. Hopeless.

Jane began working the streets at night, earning on average two dollars per customer. Some of them would pay as much as six dollars—if she was "lucky." But luck is unjust and short-lived. When morning came, she would have to surrender half of her earnings to her pimp—that same man-boy who had raped and introduced her to working the streets in the first place.

With the little earnings she had left, each morning Jane would bring food home for her family before leaving to attend her high school classes. Then at night, she would return to the brothel, and the vicious cycle would start all over again.

But, even in the darkness, Jane saw a glimmer of hope, however faint, in pursuing her academic dreams. Taking shelter in that tiny ray of light and hope, she continued to work the streets at night to pay for her first two years of high school education.

"Some customers even pay to beat you up," Jane recalled, "and one night, a man did. I was beaten so badly until my friend came in to rescue me. Bruised and bleeding, I knew I had to get out. Encouraged by another woman who had left, I also left that life behind me—finally."

Jane's story is almost beyond comprehension. After our visit, as I tried to scrub the dirt out of my clothes, a litany of difficult questions flashed through my mind: What would I do if I had the opportunity to make "easy" money, if it were the only option left for me to achieve my educational dreams? The repetitive motion of hands scrubbing against cotton clothes caused everything in my body to ache, and I keeled over from a heavy heart and wept.

This is yet another thing that I never had to face growing up as an American teenager. I realized that I never could know—truly know—the pain, anguish, violence, and imprisonment that Jane and other young women like her have endured in order to pursue their dreams.

I had no solution for the madness of Nairobi's slums. Brothers dying and children abandoned. Teenage Jane struggling to manage insecurities, worries, threats, and anxieties such as how to put food on the table for a family of four.

I didn't have any sage advice about how best to resist the lure of "easy" money to offer Jane and other young women trapped in cycles of despair and violence, chronic hunger, food insecurity, and crushing poverty.

Perhaps, if I were forced to make such an impossible choice, I would choose the same. I soon observed that the solution would not come from me, but from the hope held within Jane. After Jane finished her first semester in university, she was top of her class. In her success, she was reminded of her value as a child of God and that she was worth more than the oppression of sexual violence that was forced on her. She found hope after sexual violence in chasing her academic dreams.

Now Jane is a bold advocate against sexual violence. She says, "My vision is to see my friends come out of sex work. I want them to see my life to know that it is possible to achieve their dreams—that they too can live with freedom." Jane has spoken publicly with groups of children who are survivors of defilement, mothers who are survivors of domestic violence, teenagers caught in the cycle of forced prostitution, fathers who are fighting for justice to come for their daughters, and all who have suffered from the hunger pains of poverty. At one particular school for girls in Kenya, I saw Jane come alive as she shared her story as a survivor of rape, forced prostitution, and gross injustice. Every school girl present in the room was able to identify with her story. They also began to recognize that this same hope that Jane experienced is there for them as well. Jane, and many of these school girls, no longer feel ashamed of hunger caused by poverty—rather, they are hungry for the hope of new possibilities.

FROM HUNGER
TO HOLISTIC HEALTH

ELIZABETH URIYO AND CHRISTOPHER DELVAILLE

A dit weighed nine pounds (four kilograms) when a child development worker from a church in his village in Timor, Indonesia, met him and registered him into Compassion's program. At nine pounds, Adit would be a healthy newborn. Adit was twenty months old.

Sadly, Adit's mother died during childbirth from complications brought about by severe anemia. Desperate for work, Adit's father fled to another island, leaving his son with his impoverished parents, who fed Adit watered-down porridge twice a day.

Adit had a lung infection and was severely malnourished during this critical time in his development, when he should have weighed twenty-two to thirty-two pounds.[1] The child development worker facilitated hospitalization and the administration of a ninety-day therapeutic feeding plan consisting of five to six daily nutritional feedings.

The risks to Adit's survival were real. Protracted hunger leads to malnutrition and stunting in children. Hunger is both physical and socioemotional. Physical pain and weakness are accompanied by feelings of anxiety about availability and accessibility of food (food insecurity), alienation, and deprivation, which adversely impact familial and social interactions.[2] In 2016, globally, 5.6 million children under five died, many from preventable causes. It is estimated that malnutrition contributed to 45 percent of these deaths.[3] During this period, 815 million people globally were food insecure and malnourished, 60 percent of whom lived in conflict-stricken countries.[4] The highest populations were in Southeast Asia (64 percent), followed by sub-Saharan Africa (30 percent), and Latin America and the Caribbean (5 percent).

The Sustainable Development Goal of achieving "zero hunger" by 2030 is inextricably linked to elimination of extreme poverty.[5] This entails agricultural transformations to double productivity and incomes of smallholder farmers, as well as improving food systems, empowering rural communities (women and men alike), investing in infrastructure, and addressing access to land, financing, and markets to build resilient communities.[6] Since over 70 percent of the world's extreme poor live in rural communities where agriculture is their livelihood and about 60 percent of food consumed in developing countries is produced on small family farms, it's imperative that investments in science and technology deliver solutions that increase productivity while protecting the environment.[7]

In 2017, the General Assembly of the United Nations agreed that a global holistic response is vital since sustainable development is unattainable without peace. In times of nationalism it's essential to address the root causes of conflict and send clear messages of hope.[8] The General Assembly emphasized the importance of using platforms that involve all segments of society (including government, religious, and scientific communities) and that recognize the role of youth and women as change agents in poverty eradication and sustainable development.[9]

Working to end holistic hunger (spiritual, physical, and socioemotional depravation) is one aspect of Compassion's programs. Adit is among two million children who are known, loved, and protected by a local Compassion church partner. The church, the triumphant bride of Christ, is God's vessel bringing hope to poor, oppressed, and abandoned children such as Adit.

Adit has responded well to treatment and today is an energetic three year old. With ongoing support, Adit continues to thrive and is on track to be among the thousands and thousands of children released from hunger and poverty to actively make positive change in their world.

In the work we do, we continue to see the value of leveraging relationships to mobilize local churches, strengthening their capacity to end hunger and release children from poverty, in Jesus' name! So, we invite you to labor with us, for the harvest is plentiful, but the workers are few.

PART 3

A WAY FORWARD:
WHAT WE
CAN DO

NAME: Rupa

AGE: 19

LOCATION: Kathmandu, Nepal

When I was two years old and living in Lalitpur in the Kathmandu Valley, my father died from HIV/AIDS, and my mother was also its victim. (My biological mother is still alive, but is now in the end stages of the disease.)

After our father died, people around us, including my relatives, thought that my sister, Deepa, who was maybe four years old at the time, and I also were diagnosed with HIV/AIDS even though we were not. In the context of Nepal—and I think even in some other places around the world—HIV/AIDS is considered a curse rather than a disease.

They thought we were cursed along with our parents. Nobody wanted us. And when our father died, we were abandoned by our relatives and our neighbors. We were left alone. I don't know how we ate or if we had any food at all. I'm sure we were hungry, but I was too young to have that memory.

But I know that's how my life was.

I don't remember being turned out on the street because I was too little then. But we were by ourselves for some time before someone heard about our father, Gautham, and we were brought here to Kathmandu. (Rupa has lived with her adoptive parents, Gautham and Rekha, in the city of Kathmandu for nearly seventeen years.)

Since then we've had everything we've needed.

We didn't have to suffer physical needs, but emotionally we have suffered. Being from that kind of background, people around us have lots of questions. They judge us based on our past life. Facing people and their questions was kind of a fear for me.

The truth about my biological parents and what my life used to be became my biggest fear in facing other people. But my family has given me the strength to get around that, and now I have.

Currently I am an intern with an international NGO, Tiny Hands, that works with children who are living on the streets. Tiny Hands provides basic needs and education for the children, most of whom don't have parents. Some of them are picked up off of the streets; some of them have been abandoned by their families and have no one to take care of them. I work among them right now.

A few months ago, on the way to school I found a boy who was begging around for food. He said he was hungry and that he hadn't eaten in many days. Many people were just passing by him, and he was just shouting, but nobody was answering.

I felt bad, so I asked him what happened, and he said, *I haven't eaten for days*. At that time, I didn't have any money with me, but I searched in my bag and found some chocolates, so I gave him those. The next day, near a big bus stop in Kathmandu, I found the same boy—he was maybe nine or ten years old—asking around for food. He was saying over and over again, "I have not eaten for many days and I am very hungry; please give me something to eat."

You could see that he was dirty and wearing rags. He was begging for food, going from person to person, asking for money or food. I called to him, but I didn't want to give him money because I wasn't sure whether he would spend it on good things or bad things. He might go and buy drugs or cigarettes. So, I told him, if you're hungry just come with me. He did, and I took him to a small shop and bought him some donuts. That day, I was able to help him. Since then, I haven't seen him, but maybe I was just too busy and didn't notice him. That was my encounter with him.

Usually, children on the street are compelled to steal, because not everyone will offer them food or help. If it's just a small thing, they will get a scolding from the shopkeeper. But if they are doing it regularly, then the shopkeeper might use a hand or a stick to beat the boys and girls who are stealing.

If it's not a beating—if the case is more serious and they are stealing something expensive, the shopkeeper might call the police and hand them over. Then I think they are kept in jail for a few days. But in Nepal, if you don't have your parents and you don't have food and are left on the street, some of the boys, for instance, will say it's better to be in jail than to be on the streets, moving around all the time, begging for food. In jail, they say, at least they feed you. In jail you get a meal.

We don't have to do something big or undertake a huge project to help children like that boy who are alone and starving. We can do simple, ordinary things with extraordinary passion and love. If you have the passion to help somebody, and it's really deep, and if you are doing it out of love, even if you just give him a simple thing like a packet of biscuits, it means a lot for him.

The other thing I want to say is if we just give them food for today—here's another charity person giving us something to eat—they won't feel blessed having it. But if you do the same thing with love, it might give them a new hope. *We are special, and somebody cares for us.* They can have that feeling. And I think when they have that feeling it's more for life.

It's like that saying, "If you give a man a fish, he'll eat for a day. But if you teach the man how to fish, you feed him for a lifetime." If we give them some sort of hope that they are special and loved and cared for, it might give them a new hope for a new start.

It's not just a biscuit or a meal. It's hope, and a biscuit, and a meal.

WHEN YOU EAT,
SIT DOWN

RICK BAYLESS

I was born into a restaurant family in Oklahoma, and from the time I was very young, I worked in our restaurant and was super interested—and still am—in culture. When I got a little older, I fell in love with Mexico, which led me to do studies in language.

My undergrad degree is in Spanish-language literature and Latin American studies, and I went to graduate school to study anthropology and linguistics, the relationship between language and culture. While there, lots of my friends did field work in different places around the world, and one of my closest friends was working for a literacy organization in the highlands of Guerrero, the state next to Oaxaca in southern Mexico. It was an experience I had in Mexico that made me confront and think about the harsh realities of poverty and hunger, and was perhaps the first time I had witnessed them face to face.

The project my friend was working on in Guerrero involved codifying the Mixtec language, which at that time had never been written down. She was writing the grammar, writing the lexicon, doing basic literacy work to teach them to read and write their own language, and to begin to record some of their stories—to write them down—in Mixtec. In 1979, my wife, Deann, and I went to visit her on our honeymoon, which was a journey of what felt like ten thousand miles by bus through Mexico (and we're still married forty years later!), in a little town called Jalapa, Guerrero. From there we walked two hours into the village where she was working on her project. Our friend was also a registered nurse, so she brought a lot of supplies with her, because the villagers didn't have any kind of clinic or medical services anywhere around them.

When we finally reached the village, she told us the first thing we had to do was go around to all the people who lived there and say hello to them, one by one. As we approached the first home, she hollered from a distance that we were coming and stood there until she heard something back—just in case they had their dogs on alarm and that sort of stuff—and then we progressed to where the people were living.

When we got to one home, the people said, "Oh, please come in. We will get you some food." They *always* offer you food. So, the woman of the house went into her kitchen to prepare us something to eat, while others gathered these small chairs—their chairs are much lower than our chairs—for us to sit on while we received the food.

As I lowered myself to the chair, the woman returned. All that she had in her house at that moment was an egg. A single egg. She scrambled it, put salt on it, divided it into three parts, and offered it to us. Not only was that the most generous thing anybody has ever done for me in my entire life, it also made me realize just how close to the edge of sustenance they were living.

There was such a fine line between health and starvation for them. They lived in such a remote and rural place, that if they have a crop failure, they just basically starve until the next season. They work on a barter economy in those small villages, and so if they don't have anything to barter with, they just have to deal with what they can deal with, go out into the forest, and try to collect stuff they can eat from the wild. Man, when you look at that, it's crazy.

So that was one encounter that has stayed with me all these years.

•   •   •

The second one was here in Chicago, the only time I have ever served on a jury. There was a woman on our jury who had been raised in Cabrini-Green, the infamous high-rise public housing complex that used to sprawl across the city's Near North Side. The Chicago Housing Authority built the Frances Cabrini Row-houses and William Green Homes between 1942 and 1962, and at their peak in the 1980s, more than fifteen thousand people called the 3,600 mid-level and high-rise apartments that comprised the complex home.

By that time, Cabrini-Green essentially had become the poster-child for everything wrong with public housing in the United States. It resembled a high-rise prison, with boarded-up and burned-out windows, balconies fenced in to keep residents from throwing garbage to the ground below (or from falling or being thrown to their deaths), and concrete everywhere. Rampant crime, gang violence, drug abuse, and deplorable living conditions earned it a reputation as one of the worst places to live in Chicago, if not the entire country. The city began knocking Cabrini-Green down in 1995, and the last of its buildings was razed in 2011.

The woman on our jury had been born and raised in Cabrini. She said she had never had a job, no one in her family had ever had a job, and that the only income the family had was from the Department of Children and Family Services (DCFS)—government assistance they received based on how many kids they had.

Now, there was another African American woman on our jury who obviously didn't quite understand the woman from Cabrini-Green or her experience. The second woman lived on the city's South Side and was a very middle-class woman. She had worked at Jewel (a local chain of grocery stores in Chicago and parts of the Midwest) for twenty years, running the flower department. She was into beauty and making things beautiful. The way she described it, hers was a pretty simple existence, but beauty was important to her, and she talked about how it didn't take much to make things more beautiful.

Over a two-day trial and deliberations, there was an ongoing conversation between these two women. They were both African American and could talk to each other in a way that I could not. If I had tried to ask the woman from Cabrini questions about her life, it would have been like a newspaper reporter saying "What do you do with this? Or what do you do when that happens?" But the conversation between the two women unfolded naturally, and I just sat there quietly most of the time, listening to them. One exchange was, for me, particularly memorable.

The woman from the South Side asked the woman from Cabrini, "Do you cook for your family?"

And the woman from Cabrini said, "Oh no, I don't know how to cook."

Then the South Side woman said, "What do you serve? You could just go into the grocery store and buy some stuff and cook it."

"That sounds way too hard for me," the Cabrini woman said.

"Well, what do you have for your kids?" the South Side woman asked.

"Well, maybe once a week or something I'll buy a box of cereal and a jug of milk, and then they can have that. But I just give them a dollar and I tell them to go eat at a restaurant. If they're hungry, they just go eat at a restaurant. And they usually get some food at school," the Cabrini mother said.

There are layers of desperation in what she described. It's important also to remember that this was during the days when fast-food restaurants had those "dollar meals" on their menus. Kids could just go hand their dollar to the people behind the register and say, "Give me a dollar's worth," and they would give them whatever. And that was what they got to eat. At the time, there were fast-food restaurants all

around Cabrini. In fact, as is often the case with economically de-
pressed communities, fast-food restaurants were pretty much the *only*
restaurants in the neighborhood around Cabrini. We call them *food
deserts* now.

What struck me listening to that conversation between two Chicago
mothers was that the mom from Cabrini never expressed the idea that
someone had cooked for her when she was a child. I thought that was
interesting, because most of us have grown up with someone preparing food for us at some point.

That's why we do a lot of slow-cooker recipes in my books and
kitchens. People say, "Why so many slow-cooker recipes?" Because it's
the thing that reminds you of what it smelled like when your mom
was cooking, or your grandma was cooking or an aunt or somebody
was cooking for you, and you walked into the house and you smelled
that smell. So, I want to re-create that. Even if you have to work all day
long, you can walk in and your kids are gonna say, "Wow, she was
cooking for us today." And they're going to have that same memory
someday that you have now. Even though you started the slow-cooker
at eight o'clock in the morning, you're reaping the rewards of it when
you get home. And it's just wonderful. There's nothing like that smell
or that flavor. As I listened to the woman from Cabrini, years back, I
was so sad that she could never give that to her kids and that it was
never given to her either.

Those are the two stories that always come to my mind when I'm
asked about hunger and food insecurity. And to be in the middle of
two such different worlds—one of them out in this really impoverished rural world and then the other one in downtown Chicago—yet
the desperation was palpable in both places. That makes me stop and
think about what and how I eat. It makes you stop.

And that's connected to the thing that I always say about cooking
and about food: *when you eat, sit down.*

Sit down because that's going to make you pay attention to what you're eating. Sit down because it will slow you down. Even if it's just a little taco with some black beans, and a sprinkling of cheese over it and a spoonful of salsa, you'll recognize how special that is. And it'll just stop you for a minute, and you'll understand, and be grateful for what you have. How we eat is as important as what we eat. It's the shoving of the food in your mouth that upsets your stomach, and it doesn't connect you to the food in a way that you need to be connected to it.

●   ●   ●

To live and work in a society that throws away most of its food—I find that crazy and horrifying. I grew up with very little and have always made the most out of everything I've ever had. And it's hard for me to waste anything. Like the other night, my daughter, who lives next door to me, came over and was cooking dinner for us. I came home from work later, and she had made this nice dinner. She had made too much salad dressing by about three tablespoons. But it was made with really nice balsamic vinegar and olive oil, and she was just going to throw it away because it didn't look to her like a savable amount.

I said, "Oh, no! I can do lots of stuff with that." So, I put it away and, lo and behold, two nights later, I just needed a little bit of salad dressing, and it was perfect! But for people who are not raised thinking about every little bit of everything, it's very hard to get into that way of thinking. Meanwhile there are people in the world—in tiny rural towns in Mexico and even in our own town, in Chicago—who would love to have something like that. It would be so special to them.

There are people there and people here who are dying because they don't have enough to eat. And for us—we have so much of it we can just say, "Oh, throw it in the trash."

I don't know how we bring these two worlds together. But we have to start somewhere. Even if it's three tablespoons at a time.

•   •   •

Now, there are also big things we can do to make big changes culturally that will make a difference when it comes to fighting hunger in the world.

Number one: we need to stop thinking of food as a commodity. Food is not a commodity. Food is lifeblood.

Next, we have to stop eating in front of the television. We have to actually sit and have the moment—even if it's fifteen minutes—to connect with other human beings, with food in front of us, and where we all recognize that this moment is important, for many, many reasons. Let's sit down and look at each other and have a conversation and eat, and it doesn't have to be a big deal. Just sitting at a table connecting with another human being could be a good start.

Another thing that is important as we talk about hunger issues: learn how to cook.

If you learn to cook, then you can more adequately use what you have. My daughter doesn't know how to cook well enough, so she'll say, "I wouldn't have saved that because I wouldn't know what to do with just a little bit of it." And I might say, "Well, I can tell you three things to do with it." But she doesn't have enough experience cooking to do that because her generation just doesn't cook that much. Everything's disposable.

I think that if we are more conscientious about our food, we will be conscientious about people who don't have any. And we'll think about supporting efforts that help those people who don't have enough to get what they need. Of course, that is a very complex issue and has to do with all kinds of things that go into the governmental realm and so forth. But nevertheless, if you become more aware of your food, you'll support things that are about making access to food more equitable for everyone.

• • •

Sustainability is an important part of this discussion. But when you're just starting out, it can seem like an overwhelming issue for the average person. It may be helpful to think about it this way: sustainability starts with how you take care of yourself. So, first, take care of yourself, and then start to think a little beyond that.

A next step might be thinking about whether you should buy organic foods. Well, what does organic mean? Even though I grew up in the sixties, I did not come from the organic movement. When I started buying from local farmers because they had the stuff I wanted, it was the local farmers who taught me about sustainability. The first local farmer we really connected with and started working with a lot said to me one day, "I'm not a tomato farmer or a zucchini farmer—I'm a dirt farmer."

She taught me about how the earth, if you treat it well, will give you amazing things. But you must treat it *really* well. So, you start to think of sustainability in those terms: Well, what's best for the earth? What's best for the planet? What's in it? What's best for my body? All of those things. Then you start to think about how much you should eat. What kinds of things should you have in your diet? Where should they come from? How did they grow that stuff? Was it good? Did they just take all the nutrients out of the soil, or did they put back what needs to be in the soil for the next harvest of things?

When you're thinking about sustainability, you're thinking about all of those kinds of questions. Start with *what's going to make me healthy?* and extrapolate out from there. *What makes the world*

*healthy? What makes the guests in our restaurant healthy? What makes
our staff healthy?*

Your body, or your being, if you will, is like a microcosm of the way
you think about everything else. The issues are just too big to come
at them from the global perspective. I say it's best to start with yourself
and do something for yourself, and then the next step will come after
that, and next after that, and so on.

●　　●　　●

In our restaurant, only 5 percent of our garbage is disposed of in
a landfill.

I hear people say, "Oh, I don't think I could ever do it." And I tell
them, well, we couldn't either if we hadn't taken the first one hundred
fifty steps before we got to where we are now. We didn't start with only
5 percent. We started by asking, years ago, if we could find somebody
to pick up our glass because I don't want it to wind up in a landfill. So,
we did. We found someone to take the glass, and the glass led to card-
board, and that led to aluminum, and so on.

The next big thing was, how can we compost? Then we found
this guy just by my throwing the question out there, saying, "God,
I wish I could compost." And if you say that for long enough, somebody's going to come back to you with, "I have a solution for you: I
was at this other thing and this guy says he composts and he said
he's about ready to take on a restaurant. Do you want to work
with him?"

And I said, "Yep."

But you have to take the first step—just one little step. And then
you have to jump in with both feet. If it doesn't work out, at least you
tried it. But if it does, look where you might be and what you might
do. In our experience, it did work out—with lots of problems along

the way. But the problems were solvable. And now we can say that 95 percent of our waste stream is disposed of outside of landfills.

If you asked me what's the one step practically anybody could take that might lead to the next hundred steps that make real change in the world, I would say, go to a farmer's market. It's the vibrancy of the food in a farmer's market and the fact that most of them are out of doors, which is the place where food always tastes better because your senses are heightened when you're outdoors. Go to a farmer's market, and the food will seduce you, inspire you, and give you the power you need to overcome obstacles.

Go to the farmer's market, meet the farmers who grow the food—buy something, take it home, and cook it. It will give you a whole sense of crafting our nutrition, our sustenance. It's crafted by one person, passed to another, who crafts it, and then gives it to some other people who ingest it, and then that's their sustenance. You start to feel connected and enthusiastic about it.

Connecting with people who grow your food can be a really formative experience for people, and will give you that enthusiasm you need to take the next step after that: grow something yourself—that's a craft too. Maybe it's just a pot of herbs that you put outside your back door. Keep that one basil plant alive and use it, cook with it, put a pinch of it on your pasta.

It can be invigorating. And that will be life-giving.

BEGIN WITH LOVE

RACHEL MARIE STONE

Eating (and cooking, and procuring food) with a compassionate awareness of global hunger begins, as all good things do, with love.

By *love* I do not mean sentimentality, or romance, or pity, or affection. I mean the solid conviction that one's life is equal in worth to the life of every other person on the planet—an unshakeable commitment to offering every other human being exactly the same respect and dignity one wishes and seeks for oneself.

This may seem an odd way to begin, but if love is, as I believe, at the root of all justice and all beauty, the lack of love is at the root of all injustice and all ugliness. That some go hungry—and die of hunger—in a world that has the resources to end hunger, is unjust and ugly, and can only mean that somehow, somewhere, some of us have decided that some people deserve to be fed more than others.

Of course, no one—or nearly no one—wants to be heard stating the matter so coldly and nakedly. It is hard to live with one's conscience if one states outright, "I deserve to be fed better than *that* person," or "What *my* child eats is more important than what any other child eats." So we create abstractions and justifications that repackage these ugly ideas into stories we can live with: stories, for example, about how feeding the hungry actually exacerbates their suffering, or about how imaginary invisible hands must be left alone to do their work in "the market."

We humans tend to respond empathically when confronted, face to face, with an actual person in need. But we humans are also very, very good at creating abstractions; at telling ourselves stories that help us live with the ugliness and injustice in the world. If we actually want to make the world a little better, and not simply to assuage our own uneasy consciences, we have to resist the urge to relax into the first story that makes us feel okay about hunger in the world and our role in ending it.

If you, like me, are an educated, middle- to upper-class North American, you probably, like me, need to practice being uncomfortable with your place in the world and with the privilege you have when it comes to food.

How to begin? Again, with love: recognize that every person on this planet is, fundamentally, more *like you* than *not like you*, and that, just as you wish for yourself and your loved ones to be well fed and well loved, so it is with *all people*. When citizens and policymakers forget this, we begin to justify the unjustifiable, and we fail to treat our global neighbors as we would wish to be treated.

THE QUESTIONS TO ASK

We must remember that people who are poor and people who experience hunger and malnutrition in its various forms (in the United States, obesity rates are high among those who are poor, and the diets of people with low incomes are often abysmally deficient in nutrients) are just like everyone else in their needs and desires. If we forget this, we are in danger of hurting or condescending to others even when our intentions are good. If we begin with love, we can hope to help in ways that nurture human dignity and flourishing in all of its beautiful variety. If we do not, we run the risk of imposing our own sense of

How Things Ought To Be on others. Well-meaning people often have harmed unintentionally where they meant to help because they have forgotten to cultivate this humility.

Here is a nonedible example: years ago, I helped with a mitten drive at an affluent preschool. The vast majority of the donations were the sort of cheap, dollar-store, synthetic stretch gloves that begin to pill and unravel almost as soon as they're worn. None of the children who attended the preschool actually wore cheap gloves like that. I was surprised, then, when one mother showed up with several pairs of children's mittens from the same high-end store from which most of her son's clothes came. I thanked her for her generosity, exclaiming at the quality of her gift. "It's for charity," she shrugged. "I wouldn't want to give something cheap."

Hers is the attitude to emulate: *What sort of mittens would I put on my child's hands? What sort of food would I pack in my daughter's lunch?*

Ask yourself these sorts of questions: *How would I want food assistance policy to be implemented if I were going to need it? What would be the most dignified and life-giving way to offer and to receive food assistance? What sort of food pantry or soup kitchen experience would feed me in body and soul, and leave me feeling respected and honored?*

It is easy to think that people who find themselves needing to seek help will be endlessly grateful for day-old pastry or off-brand peanut butter or boxed macaroni and cheese. But even people in extreme need have the same sorts of preferences as you and I, preferences for food that is fresh, wholesome, tasty, culturally and nutritionally appropriate, familiar, nourishing, and delivered with dignity and respect.

PRACTICING NONJUDGMENTAL CURIOSITY

I believe that cultivating respect for other people includes cultivating respect for their foodways, and that, in a family, this should begin in childhood and continue as a lifelong discipline. That is, taste promiscuously, and, if you are a parent, expose your children to a variety of foods and food traditions, and make it a matter of principle not to judge others on any grounds for what they eat or don't eat.

It is natural, of course, to feel distaste, or even disgust, for unfamiliar foods. That is why ethnic slurs, not infrequently, include references to the characteristic culinary habits of the slandered group. (In the film *It's a Wonderful Life*, the greedy and unfeeling Mr. Potter dismisses the generosity of the Bailey Building & Loan toward the immigrant community by alleging that the Baileys "play nursemaid to a bunch of garlic-eaters.") A standard complaint about immigrant and refugee families in apartment buildings is that their cooking smells "strange" or "stinks," and persecution of Muslims, Jews, Hindus, and others have often included the derogation and desecration of their respective sacred food prohibitions.

The opposite of this would be *xenophilia*—love and affection for that which is "foreign" or "different." In every culture, sharing food is shorthand for sharing friendship, and expressing interest in the foods of someone else's region, country, or culture can be a powerful gesture of friendship and love.

International Night is one of the most joyful events of the year at the boarding school where I live and teach. Our students, who represent many different countries and cultures, set up food stalls offering small portions of signature dishes and drinks. It means a lot to students when their teachers taste kimchee or haggis or pierogi or goat curry or plantains and pronounce it "good." It means something very close to *I accept you as you are*, or even, *I love you.*

You might ask your friends and coworkers about their favorite foods, or the foods that they grew up with, especially if their background is different from yours. Visit the sort of ethnic restaurants that are patronized mostly by people of that particular ethnicity, and ask for recommendations. If none of this is accessible to you, commit to tasting your way through a variety of global cuisines by using an international cookbook such as *Extending the Table* or *The Best International Recipe*.

Your church or community group could host a potluck or community supper in the spirit of International Night. The goal is not merely to cultivate cosmopolitan tastes but rather to find common ground with others, overcoming food prejudice and underscoring shared human experience.

Don't allow your children—or yourself—to express disgust at others' food habits. Encourage them to say, instead, "I don't care for XYZ" rather than "XYZ *is gross.*" Don't air your judgments about other people's diets. Instead, seek understanding and a nonjudgmental attitude. Perhaps the person buying only ice cream and pudding is bringing it to a dying relative who no longer can swallow anything else. You don't know all there is to know.

Offer presumptive respect when it comes to differences of all kinds, including social and economic class differences. Don't assume you know how poor white Southerners eat, or how rural Mainers eat, or how Afro-Caribbean New Yorkers eat. Don't ridicule how *anyone* eats. Everyone has a story that you have not yet learned.

MORE THAN "A PERSONAL CHOICE"

I began with love because it is important to reject the idea that what we eat is entirely a matter of personal preference and private choice. Eating is both intensely inward and personal (digestion is about as inward and as personal as you can get), and at the same time, eating is connected to plants, animals, soil, weather, and, of course, people, politics, culture, and history. For most of human history, people either gathered, killed, or grew most of what they ate, or knew the people who did. By contrast, last week at a rest stop, I saw a bag of trail mix containing ingredients from six different countries.

The idea that what an individual or family eats—or doesn't eat—can have an impact on ecology and on world hunger has been around for a while. Frances Moore Lappe's *Diet for a Small Planet* (1971) and Doris Janzen Longacre's *More-With-Less* cookbook (1977) prompted people to think differently about the giant slabs of meat that post-World War II prosperity (and synthetic nitrogen fertilizers and burgeoning factory farms) had plunked down on their plates relatively cheaply. Meat—especially beef—they argued, exacted costs beyond the price-per-pound. Its production disproportionately consumed resources of land, water, and fossil fuels and thus represented waste. These writers framed overconsumption in wealthy countries as directly connected to famine in other countries, investing dietary choices with social and moral import.

These books, and many others that followed (including, notably, Michael Pollan's *The Omnivore's Dilemma* in 2006) helped catapult the ethics of eating to the front of many consumers' consciousness. Along with the ever-evolving awareness of health considerations, food has become invested with a sense of moral importance that North Americans of all faith and no faith could embrace, and, predictably, clever marketers have come along to bathe their brands in a morally superior light.

Walk into any Whole Foods and you'll see what I mean: many brand names are loaded with moral import, with words such as "pure," "honest," "caring," and "innocent" gracing the labels. "Guilt" and "conscience" are frequently invoked, and, often, the environmental impact of the product or its packaging also is indicated on the label. Whether these claims of moral superiority are warranted is up for debate.

Whole Foods, not incidentally, has been dubbed popularly "Whole Paycheck," and shopping there, as opposed to, say, a deep-discount chain, has become something of a status-marker—a signal of eco- and health-conscious consumerism that is way out of reach for many

North American families, let alone hungry people in the Majority World. It would be a mistake, then, to buy into the feel-good stories that places such as Whole Foods evoke and consider that we have done our duty when it comes to food justice.

Just as the gospel is not actually the gospel unless it is "good news for the poor," food is neither "pure" nor "innocent" nor "guilt-free" unless it, in some way, participates in a system that ameliorates hunger or environmental degradation, and promotes flourishing and true wholeness.

Full disclosure: I shop at Whole Foods (not exclusively, but I do). But I don't frame it as a moral virtue, however much the marketing tempts me to do so.

WASTE LESS AND SIMPLIFY

I'm not just talking about table scraps. Experts have estimated that as much as half of the food that's grown in the United States is wasted. When you consider all the resources of time, energy, water, human labor, and more that go into producing food, the ugliness of waste seems all the more apparent, particularly in light of global hunger. Commit to cutting your family's food waste in half. Buy smaller amounts, freeze things before they spoil, learn to love leftovers, pause before you order takeout, eliminate all things disposable. Simply becoming a little more conscious of waste reduces your environmental impact while also saving you a few dollars that can be put toward reputable charities that work to eliminate hunger.

If you do not cook from scratch, begin to do so. In 2016, Herald Press released a revised edition of *More-With-Less*. I had the privilege of working on the revisions in consultation with others, and one of our aims was to make the instructions even more accessible to readers with minimal kitchen experience. *More-With-Less* is a primer on simple, thrifty cooking from scratch, and, if you are reliant on takeout, prepared foods, and heavily meat-centric meals, undoubtedly will save you money. Many of the recipes can be prepared in less time than it takes to go out to eat. Again, you might find that it frees up some money that you can put toward the cause of alleviating hunger.

POLICY, POLICY, POLICY

By all means, "vote with your fork," as the foodies say, but pay attention to policy as well. Does the Farm Bill respect human flourishing in all aspects, including by protecting the fragile resources of soil and water? Do public assistance policies degrade those who seek help in putting food on the table? Do foreign-aid and trade bills guard against greed and promote sustainable practices?

Apply the love test: *If I were the person directly affected by this policy, how would I wish to be treated?* Recognize that these matters often are highly complicated, but also recognize that high levels of "complication" often are invoked to cloak inhumane ugliness, injustice, and greed. Be skeptical of easy fixes and comforting stories.

FIGHT THE LONG DEFEAT

Paul Farmer, the remarkable humanitarian doctor and the soul behind Partners in Health, acknowledges the seemingly insurmountable obstacles he and his partners are up against in fighting, for example, treatment-resistant tuberculosis, and offers wisdom for those who, like us, want to be victorious over injustice:

"What we're really trying to do in [Partners in Health] is to make common cause with the losers," Farmer writes. "We want to be on the winning team, but at the *risk* of turning our backs on the losers, no, it's not worth it. So, you fight the long defeat."

It would be hubris, of course, to think we could end hunger in our time by our individual efforts alone. But if it were *your* child who was hungry, you would try.

Love bids us to fight the long defeat.

END HUNGER

Do the Thing That's in Front of You

TONY P. HALL

T*ony, isn't it time* to bring God into your workplace?"

Members of Congress are buffeted constantly with an ever-rushing river of facts, opinions, politics, and legislation. In the handful of years I had been in Congress before hearing this life-changing question, both supportive and angry constituents had confronted me with tough questions about the positions I held on a multitude of issues, from farm subsidies and transportation bills to naming post offices and military funding at the height of the Cold War.

But no question had been more unsettling than the one a friend and mentor asked me early in my congressional career: "Tony, isn't it time to bring God into your workplace?"

Through a good portion of my adult life, I had not considered myself a strong man of faith by any means. In fact, it was not until after I entered Congress that a strong sense of spiritual conviction took a guiding role in my life. Even so, I was never comfortable wearing my faith on my lapel the way that some of my congressional colleagues did. I often tell people that I would rather see a sermon than hear one, and in my own life I would rather act out my faith than preach it. This is still the case.

Over the years I have learned that bringing God into the workplace is not a goal in and of itself. It is a means to understanding how I can do my small part in realizing the capital-U Ultimate goal of bringing the kingdom to the world.

My continuing journey to bring God into the workplace has focused extensively if not exclusively on my passion to end hunger around the world. The following anecdotes paint a picture of how my understanding of the issue of hunger has evolved through the lenses of faith, politics, and current issues.

VALLEY OF THE SHADOW OF DEATH

My first visit to Ethiopia was life changing. In 1984, I traveled to Ethiopia on a fact-finding mission in my capacity as chair of the International Hunger subcommittee of the House Select Committee on Hunger. My trip coincided with the height of a devastating famine in that country, and what I witnessed was nothing short of earth-shattering.

On one excursion, I was traveling with a group of medical professionals to an internally displaced persons camp. This camp was "home" to thousands of Ethiopians seeking safe haven from civil war, as well as from one of the worst periods of drought the country had seen in modern history. While at the camp, we stopped at a medical facility where the sheer weight of human distress was suffocating. I still find it difficult to convey the pure sensory overload that accompanies this kind of scene.

It was a hunger you could see. A hunger you could hear and smell. A hunger you could almost taste.

Mothers, spotting the white foreigner, assumed that I was a doctor and would hand their children to me. Often, there was nothing left to be done for these children. Sometimes the children were already dead. The tragedy deepened as I learned that many of these women already had made the impossible choice to leave a dying child behind on the road to the camp and continue the journey, realizing if they didn't, none of their children or family members would make it.

I watched two dozen children die that day. For the people at that camp, despair was the only rational response.

But I realized two things that would set me on a course for the rest of my career. First, despite how bad the environmental conditions were in Ethiopia, descending into famine was avoidable. If a drought like the one in Ethiopia had occurred in the United States, or Canada, or France, we would not have seen the need for camps like the one I visited. There was a civil war in Ethiopia at the time, so political attention and money was focused—sometimes willfully—away from these people, and toward military conquests. Famine, I learned, was not the result of a lack of food, but a lack of political will to care.

Second, on my flight home I realized that doing something about all of this was how I was going to bring God into my work.

Some years later I was once again in the same region that seems to be unable to unshackle itself from war, hunger, and injustice. A friend and I were standing outside a desolated village in the northern region of southern Sudan. The country was locked in the turmoil of war, with paramilitary groups inciting terror among civilian populations, and this village had been destroyed by self-declared Mujahideen forces from northern Sudanese regions. After inspecting the village my friend turned to me and, referencing Psalm 23, said, "This truly is the valley of the shadow of death." I thought back on what I had witnessed years earlier in Ethiopia and looked at the ruins of the village in front of me. Such a small part of the world with so much suffering. How could we hope to make any difference in this sea of tragedy?

A tiny woman a continent away had the answer.

THE THING THAT'S IN FRONT OF US

No single person has influenced how I approach the intersection of faith, poverty, and hunger quite like Mother Teresa. Her tremendous contributions to the poor in Kolkata sent waves throughout the world, and for many people, her name is synonymous with faithful humanitarian outreach.

I had the great privilege of meeting Mother Teresa on multiple occasions in India, and hers was a significant influence on my journey to bring God into my work. I will never forget the very first time I met her—after introducing myself, she took my hand in hers and, gripping each of my fingers one by one and folding them into my palm, she said, "For. The. Least. Of. These."

It is easy to get caught up in the daily grind of congressional life. As a member of Congress who also was a person of faith, I constantly struggled to reground myself in my spiritual convictions. One way I did this was through prayer time with colleagues and friends, but sometimes all it took was a simple reminder of the true love in which my faith needs to be rooted. Mother Teresa, in that one action, provided me with a memory that helped me stay focused on one of the great universal laws: to love my neighbors as myself. This was just the first experience I had with her.

Of all the memorable visits I had with Mother Teresa, one remains most vivid in my mind. By this time, I had been to Ethiopia, and the desolation and suffering caused by its famine still were stark in my memory. One day, as I watched Mother Teresa at work amid a throng of poor and hungry people in Kolkata (what appeared to be an endless and sometimes thankless job), I remembered the scenes in Ethiopia and how the seemingly endless work that needed to be done there left me feeling futile. Considering this, I asked Mother Teresa whether she had any advice for those confronted by so much pain and suffering.

She looked at me and said, simply, "You do the thing that's in front of you."

This simple yet profound piece of advice became my mantra. As a congressman, the things that were in front of me were more than paying lip service to the poor or volunteering in a soup kitchen. They included legislation and political clout. This simple, powerful story has never been lost on me, and I still share it frequently in articles, op-eds, and speeches.

ADVERSITY

One of the most challenging and disappointing moments of my career came, unsurprisingly, from the US Congress. In the early-1990s, as part of a drive for congressional fiscal belt-tightening, Congress de-funded the House Select Committee on Hunger. This is when it really struck me that hunger was not a priority for our nation's political leaders. From that point forward, I committed myself to building the will to end hunger by making the issue more of a political priority. My faith helps to drive this mission, as it did my response to the elimination of the Hunger Committee.

Following the defunding of the Select Committee on Hunger, I decided I would fast until I felt confident that the poor and hungry would not be forgotten by Congress. As I mentioned earlier, I am uncomfortable wearing my faith as a badge and professing it publicly, so you might imagine how uncomfortable the thought of fasting as a congressman made me feel. But it was "the thing that's in front of me."

I ended up fasting for twenty-two days. The impact exceeded what I imagined it might. While I was not able to bring the Select Committee on Hunger back to fruition, the fast inspired countless people across the country to join me, including high school students, faith-based and secular organizations, churches, and even a couple of my fellow legislators. It also caught the attention of the World Bank, which responded to the fast with a $100 million commitment to fund microfinance initiatives in impoverished communities worldwide. Muhammad Yunis, the head of microloan-specializing Grameen Bank and one of the beneficiaries of the commitment, estimates that initial $100 million in microloans over time has grown to $500 million.

By getting out of my comfort zone, staying strong in my faith, and doing the thing in front of me, I was able to wake a few people up to the issue of hunger and even make a small difference for at least a few hungry families in the world.

SO WHAT? FAITH AND ENDING HUNGER
IN THE TWENTY-FIRST CENTURY

The stories above shine a light on the personal experiences that drove my passion to eliminate hunger from the world. They also highlight the critical role faith has played in shaping my approach to that work. I have met countless others with the same kinds of stories and convictions who work tirelessly to battle poverty, hunger, and all similar injustices in the world. For these kindred spirits, I am ever thankful.

But currently, we face a time that is trying our faith and resolve in battling global hunger. At the time of this publication, hunger—both in real numbers *and* as a proportion of the global population—is on the rise for the first time in a decade. Civil war and the insistent, growing pressures of a changing climate have sent South Sudan, Somalia, northern Nigeria, Yemen, and increasingly the Democratic Republic of the Congo spiraling into famine-like conditions. And once again, just as they did in 1980s Ethiopia, the willful decisions of politicians are killing countless people.

In my talks at churches, schools, and other groups interested in hunger around the world, I often mention that in many cases it is not actually the lack of food that kills starving people. Without proper nutrition, diseases run rampant over compromised immune systems, and sickness ends up killing the hungry before starvation does. When a man, woman, or child is hungry, diseases exploit and make quick work of these innocent victims.

From Ethiopia in the 1980s to Yemen today, I have learned that this applies to entire nations as well as individual humans. When a nation's people are starving, the violence and injustices that may have been simmering beneath the surface of a society are able to wreak havoc in a way they had not before. And either intentional policies or willful ignorance can emaciate an entire country.

So, what, as people of faith, can we do about this? How can doing what's in front of us put us on track to end global hunger for good?

Presently, I work with an organization called The Alliance to End Hunger. Its mission is to engage diverse institutions to build the public and political will to end hunger in the United States and around the world. It accomplishes this by empowering organizations, networks, and individual people on the front lines of the fight against hunger to raise their voices as advocates for those who historically have lacked a political voice of their own.

Our faith can and should drive us to do the same. Ultimately, if we mobilize our faith to build the will to end hunger, slowly but surely, we can succeed. In fact, I believe we have been directed to do just this. In Luke 10:25-37, Jesus has a conversation with a lawyer in which the lawyer recognizes that the greatest commandments are "'Love the Lord your God with all your heart and with all your soul and with all your strength and with all your mind'; and 'Love your neighbor as yourself.'" The lawyer, however, wants to know who his neighbor *is*. Jesus then tells the famous parable in which a Samaritan (a people reviled by many Jews at the time) stops to help a stranger who has been badly beaten and robbed, and who a number of other passersby ignored or refused to help. The upshot of the story is that the good Samaritan recognized the man in need as his neighbor.

The good Samaritan parable is more than a story about how nice it is to be nice to others. It's about going out of our way—and beyond our comfort zones—to "do the thing in front of us," not only for those we do not know or understand, but also for those we might consider to be "other," unworthy, or even our enemies.

How would the good Samaritan react to a single American mother of four in need of safety net support? I daresay there are many self-professed Christians who would jump to judge her life decisions and the contents of her grocery cart before they'd lift a finger to advocate on her behalf. Similarly, how would a good Samaritan approach Muslims in Yemen? Migrants in Italy and Hungary? Rohingya in Myanmar and Bangladesh? Undocumented immigrants in the United States?

In countries such as the United States and others with democratic traditions, we are in the unique position to be good Samaritans through advocacy. In an age when we turn on the television and browse the news online, we can see the hungry all around us, all the time. What would the good Samaritan in Jesus' parable do if he saw those images and read those stories? Not only *should* we use our faith to advocate to build the will to end poverty and hunger, I believe our faith *requires* us to do so.

One more note about this parable: when you consider the people listening to Jesus speak, and then consider the characters in the story he tells, you come to realize that, socially and culturally, Jesus' audience probably more closely identified with the man who was beaten than the Samaritan who helped him. If we picture ourselves as the persons in desperate need of help, who would we want our neighbors to be?

ONE MORE DROP

I have grown to learn the power of advocacy as the "thing that's in front of me" to bring about an end to hunger. It is how I bring God into my work, and I believe other people of faith can do the same. As a congressman, and later as an ambassador, I was influenced greatly by what I saw and experienced and the people I met along the way.

As people of faith and witnesses for the poor and hungry, you can urge your community and national leaders to see what you see. Invite them to a food bank or pantry. Encourage them to travel to countries in the developing world. Turn on your computer and write your legislator a simple email. You may not feel like you are doing much, but it adds up.

During one of my visits with Mother Teresa, a reporter asked her what drove her to continue her ministry, if her small acts of kindness felt like mere drops in a bucket. She responded, "No, what I do is a drop in the ocean, but if I didn't do it, it would be one less drop."

If that rationale is good enough for Mother Teresa, then it is good enough for us.

FROM THE GARDEN
TO THE TABLE

AMY GRANT

I t is so important that we understand food—the fuel we give our bodies, the sustenance that nurtures our souls. From the soil and the seed to the harvest and the cooking, food is an act of servitude we cultivate by hand and the foundation for nourishing our communities and ourselves.

On New Year's Day this year, my daughter, Sarah, and my niece, Sally Anne, announced they had a dream to create a raised-bed garden on our farm that would feed not just our family, but hopefully someday our community as well. It was a grand vision. And thankfully they have had the ingenuity and fortitude to make it work.

It's been amazing to watch their vision take shape as they have incorporated all the resources they've had on hand. Felled cedar trees on our property became lumber to build the first four raised beds. They asked their friends to donate compost and found quality heirloom seeds at our local public library's annual seed swap. Slowly and surely, their garden began to grow. Gardens are magical spaces. With just a little sunlight and rainwater, tiny seeds emerge from the earth, sprout and flower, producing fruits and vegetables—food! And so, the great harvest begins.

In addition to the abundance of beautiful, delicious produce that will be its bounty as summer turns to autumn, the girls and all of us who have worked alongside them in the garden are reaping the unexpected blessings of the experience. How easily conversation flows as we circle the beds to pull weeds. How connected we feel, body and soul, and to one another, with our hands in the dirt.

The garden is not just central to how and what we eat; it is the axis for building friendships and community. Our family is learning how to be less wasteful and manage our excess, and to discover new benefits of spending time outside in the glory of nature. Over breakfast, we wonder what vegetables might finally be ready to pick and eat in time for dinner. We think more critically about our food, including the meats, grains, vegetables, and all that we choose to purchase at our local grocery stores and restaurants. As we pay closer attention to and participate in our food production and preparation, we are reflecting more deeply on the intense effort, care, and even the spiritual practice of what and how we eat.

I have plenty. My children have plenty. But many parents and children do not.

Not everyone has access to the magic of a garden and the bounty of vitamins and minerals that fresh fruits and vegetables provide. In a world where political and military conflicts often trigger crises that include widespread famine, for millions of people, hunger is a reality—and one that means irreparable and long-term health consequences for countless mothers, babies, children, and families.

How do we stop it? How do we end hunger?

What if the answer is very simple—and totally doable?

I'm no expert on this, but I do know a thing or two about the importance of cooking. There is an art to preparing and sharing a meal around a table with family and friends that is simple, yet so life-giving. Cooking grounds me. When I would be out on the road for days or weeks at a time, the first thing I would do when I got home was head to the grocery store and start cooking. The monotonous tasks of prep work—cleaning, peeling, chopping—free my mind. In fact, there are monasteries with spiritual practices built around just these kinds of repetitive tasks. I believe there is a deep, spiritual truth to be found in the kitchen, where the rhythms and rituals of making a meal anchor me, helping to bring me back from the chaos and busy-ness of the road.

Back home after being on the road for an extended period of time, I'd make meals that would take hours to create—my secret pot roast or a big pot of vegetable soup. Volume was the key; I would make maybe five or six roasts at a time for what I called a "faith feast." With our huge family, not a morsel was wasted.

Over the years, I've kept up this practice of making faith feasts. But they're always impromptu—there's too much stress in a stressful world already to cook for a planned event, and I don't recommend it. I do, however, encourage, you to spontaneously cook a meal with maybe two or three times as much food as you need and share the meal later that day with someone else, whether it's a colleague, a friend, or somebody you just met. It's fun, builds community, and deepens friendships. It's also an act of faith: you make the meal with all the extra food believing that you will find the right people to share it with (or that they will find you).

Cooking also is an act of hospitality, welcoming people to your home and table. Never say no to a guest who asks if they can help in the kitchen. The answer is always yes. I've learned over the years that if I have something difficult to say to someone, I sit next to them, not across from them. There is a different connection, albeit subtle, being alongside someone instead of across from them, face to face. Working together in the kitchen, cooking side by side, provides that same kind of opportunity. It makes it easier to talk and easier to connect. In the kitchen, guests quickly become friends.

Ending hunger isn't just about food; it's also about forging these deep connections with family, friends, and community. Amid our current toxic political and cultural environment in the United States and elsewhere around the world, many of these relationships are broken, and many of us feel disconnected. Dinner in a three-star Michelin restaurant will leave us hungry for intimacy if we eat it in isolation. Studies have shown that there is no greater danger to our health than loneliness. It's not just an illness. It can trigger genetic changes that can cause further illness and even early death.

Hunger is about need, and that need is deeply multidimensional and multifaceted. Part of the solution to global hunger is ending loneliness. A shared table can be an answer.

A popular adage says, "Hurt people hurt people, and blessed people bless people." What if hunger, malnutrition, and food insecurity experienced in urban "food deserts" across the United States and in impoverished communities around the world are the "hurts" that give root to despair, violence, and even terrorism?

In the book of Matthew, Jesus tells his disciples, "For I was hungry and you gave me something to eat, I was thirsty and you gave me something to drink. . . . Truly I tell you, whatever you did for one of the least of these brothers and sisters of mine, you did for me" (Matthew 25:35-40). Jesus spoke often about food—crops and harvests, meals and banquets. Some of his most famous miracles involved thirsty and hungry people. Two thousand years after he turned water into wine at the wedding in Cana and fed a crowd of five thousand with only seven loaves of bread and a few fish, clean water and nutrition are two of the greatest challenges facing the world. Today, about 815 million people—10 percent of the world's population—live with chronic malnutrition,[1] and 780 million people live without access to clean drinking water.[2]

Still, Jesus calls us to meet these needs, starting with the "least of these" among us. We can begin the gospel work of ending hunger by initiating change under our own roofs and in our own kitchens.

In an age where people agree on almost nothing, it's hard to argue with feeding the hungry. Call it food love—a simple, yet profound tool to change the world, beginning with our own tables.

HUNGER, FASTING, AND FAITH

ÁNGEL F. MÉNDEZ MONTOYA

We are hungry beings. Without food we perish.

Hunger is one of the most primordial experiences of interdependence between people and the planet. Sadly, there is too much hunger in today's world. An estimated 815 million people worldwide (thirty-five million more than in 2017) currently live with hunger. Some communities—particularly in southern Sudan, Nigeria, Somalia, and Yemen—experience extreme famine. The wretched face of famine and world hunger is primarily caused by violent conflict, the planet's climatic deterioration, discrimination, and indifference.[1]

But there is more than one kind of hunger in the world. In addition to material and physical hunger, there is emotional and spiritual hunger. We hunger for recognition, for love and care. There is a hunger for justice and peace. There is even a hunger for God.

We hunger for what is other, whether a piece of bread, or another person. And, as there is hunger, there is also bread, nourishment. Food nourishes the body, but also the heart, the intellect, and the spirit. When the other nourishes us, otherness is experienced as a gift.

The other is an alimentary gift that propels me to also become a gift for the other, to become a source of nourishment. The gift for the other who physically, emotionally, or spiritually hungers becomes a gesture of caring and justice, of solidarity and nonindifference. It is fascinating to observe that for most historical religions the symbol for otherness is food. In most religious practices and rites, the sharing of food enables a celebration of being in community with people, the planet, and the divine.

It is, perhaps, because hunger and food are so fundamental that many religious rituals and practices are rooted in symbols of feasting and fasting. There is a rich wisdom and spiritual benefit when religions implicate and balance both practices. While there is a general, popular awareness about the benefits of feasting, the same is not true about the practice of fasting.

Precisely because of the urgent need to think critically about the brutal reality of hunger in today's world, I invite you to consider the importance of fasting as a means to achieve bodily, political, and spiritual awareness of the call to collaborate for the common good—particularly for those who most experience hunger.

There is a medical approach to understanding the benefits of fasting. Although scientific literature classifies a range of different types of fasting, there are two main types: the first is a fast in which neither food nor liquid are ingested for a defined period of time, and the second type is a restriction of food or calories that are consumed daily. Both kinds of fasting are meant to be carried out voluntarily.

Fasting is understood not only from a medical and scientific perspective, but also from a spiritual perspective as a practice with spiritual benefits. Fasting contributes to spiritual well-being, a kind of well-being that seeks a favorable and positive transformation, both personally and interpersonally. Here I refer to a spirituality that integrates the experience of the sacred and the symbolic, as well as a certain orientation toward transcendence.

For some people and communities, spiritual well-being is a social contract that transcends a merely private experience and seeks harmonious relations with otherness—other people, other cultural expressions and traditions, the environment and ecology, and the sacred. *Spiritual* comprises a broad range of religious traditions globally, as well as those experiences that go beyond doctrinal boundaries and are embedded in peoples, cultures, and communities throughout the planet and history. Spirituality is a life orientation that evokes a vision of the human being as a whole.

It is well known that the world's great historical religions, such as Hinduism, Buddhism, Judaism, Christianity, and Islam, have practiced fasting since ancient times. Believers throughout the world include fasting during certain important days, periods, and seasons of their religious calendars. Most religions practice fasting primarily as a form of bodily and spiritual cleansing, creating personal and communal connections with important traditions inscribed within the history of each religious group.

Within the religious world, fasting is practiced during important transitions or life-cycle events such as marking the passage from childhood to adolescence, preparing couples to celebrate wedding rites, assuming a position of leadership within a community, or initiating an important change in the life of an individual or community. Whether fasting is considered a way of cleansing or a means of preparing both the individual person and the community to go through transitions of great relevance in life, religious fasting is not only physical, but also simultaneously spiritual.

It is interesting to note that most religious practices of fasting are spiritual, but are, nonetheless, deeply corporeal. In most fasting practices in religious contexts, abstaining from food and liquid is considered a means of personal and communal purification, strengthening, and protection. It is important to highlight that fasting is never understood in an isolated or absolute way.

In a religion's many food symbolisms and practices, eating and fasting always go hand in hand. Feasting and fasting are so mutually complementary that for each expression of food sacrifice and deprivation there is also a festive equivalent, in which food ingestion occupies a privileged place in the spiritual life of both individuals and religious communities. Both eating and abstention from food and liquid carry a symbolism that according to religious traditions promotes spiritual growth and opens the necessary consciousness to attain personal, communal, ecological, and sacred-transcendent well-being.

In Christian traditions, this complementary aspect between feasting and fasting plays an important role in the believers' spiritual development. In fact, the Eucharist is a core symbol in Christian religions. In the Eucharist, the divine presence par excellence is embedded in a food symbol: God becomes food and drink in order to be divided and shared among the celebrants. The Christian Eucharist celebrates God as food as a way of inviting communities to become a form of nourishment themselves, to become a kind of Eucharist for others, above all for those who suffer physical-material and affective-spiritual hunger. It is only under this Eucharistic model that the place fasting occupies within the Christian worldview can be understood. Fasting is not carried out as an end in itself, but rather as a practice that serves to raise awareness of the many types of hunger existing in the world, seeking personal and communal transformation in order to eradicate all forms of violence.

In Christianity, fasting has biblical reminiscences. In the Judeo-Christian biblical world, fasting was mainly practiced as a symbolic act of bodily purification aimed at creating a more intimate bond between humanity and God. At the same time, it served to raise more awareness about the human community, in particular to express solidarity with those who suffer more. For this reason, the practice of fasting in Christianity is always accompanied by practices of hospitality, generosity, and charity, and the cultivation of virtues and values such as love, peace, and justice. In some Christian practices of fasting, periodic abstinence may consist of reducing the consumption of food and liquids, but also reducing excessive shopping and the massive volumes of waste and trash we produce. It may also consist of diminishing selfish attitudes and learning to share with others, above all those who are in greater need. It may also include dissolving a spirit of bitterness and isolation in order to learn the delight experienced in conviviality and the joy of celebrating with others. It is only under a comprehensive vision (fasting and feasting, individual and communal transformation, body and spirit) that fasting can be understood as contributing toward spiritual well-being.

In Christianity, fasting is reflective of a spiritual tradition in which the body is not only understood individually, but also with a sociopolitical dimension. Fasting here is understood from the perspective of food practices, particularly from the point of view of the Eucharist, in which personal and communal feasting and fasting culminate in the ingestion of God. According to Walker Bynum, religious women in the Middle Ages who carried out fasting and feasting practices even imagined the body (simultaneously personal and communal) as a theological place or divine locus.

The spiritual well-being attained through fasting also enables higher political consciousness, above all when fasting is practiced as a form of public protest through a hunger strike. In our time, during which we continue to witness the wounds of worldwide famine, fasting can strengthen a stance of resistance and protest systems that produce and perpetuate famine and malnutrition. Fasting as a form of political resistance also strengthens the desire to express solidarity with those who suffer hunger, poverty, marginalization, and vulnerability. A hunger strike is not an end in itself, since it is an expression of solidarity not only with causes that demand sociopolitical justice, but also with political proposals that favor the protection of the Earth, forests, air, water, animals, and plants in this critical time. Spiritual well-being sought through fasting practices is thus not only individual in character. It also includes the imperative of developing policies for the well-being of our entire human and planetary environment.

Finally, in this time governed by capitalism, consumerism, massive waste, perpetual media bombardment, individualism, and indifference toward others, we consider that fasting fosters spiritual well-being since it creates communal consciousness and reduces the excessive desire for consumerism at the cost of human and planetary exploitation. Fasting may also consist of abstinence from acts of violence and selfishness, mental chatter and physical noise, as well as polluting, toxic, and alienating practices. *We are what we eat*, and unfortunately our eating habits and food policies are leading to destruction, exploitation, and the extinction of human and planetary life.

For this reason, it is imperative that we see fasting as a way of encouraging physical and spiritual well-being. From a theological perspective, then, fasting is understood as encouraging spiritual well-being inasmuch as it serves to create a harmonious relationship with each other and our environment.

FEEDING THE HUNGRY
BY RAISING DIGNITY

KIMBERLY WILLIAMS-PAISLEY AND BRAD PAISLEY

*E*ditor's note: *Among the many things Kimberly Williams-Paisley and Brad Paisley have in common are the faith and values their own parents instilled in them growing up, including a responsibility to help others—particularly those Jesus described as "the least of these." That commitment to making life better for the less fortunate—especially families that don't have enough to eat—is something the Paisleys work hard to impart to their sons and hope to inspire in others.*

In the conversation that follows, the Paisleys discuss how they became involved in hunger issues, what they've taught their sons about caring for people who don't have enough to eat, and the practical actions they hope their experiences as parents and people of faith might inspire in others.

KIMBERLY: I grew up with a mother who loved to volunteer and help in our community. Although my parents often worried about money, we never wondered where our next meal was coming from. Actually, one of my earliest memories is of my mom throwing us in the back of a car and us riding around with her as she delivered Meals on Wheels.

Later she worked in the nonprofit world and turned out to be a fantastic fundraiser for several different important causes, including Parkinson's disease, cancer, and education. But my memory of her passion for service began with her addressing hunger in our community.

I was busy starting a family in Tennessee when my mother got diagnosed with dementia years later, and it was difficult to help her where she was in New York. One of the first things I did was go to Meals on Wheels locally and volunteer for a few years. Once in a while I would take my kids with me as well, mirroring what my mother did with me.

I loved Meals on Wheels because it was a great way to get to know the people I was serving. I loved seeing the same folks every time. I had a different perspective on it as a grownup. When my mom got sick, my parents actually could've qualified for Meals on Wheels. They didn't reach out for that kind of help, but they could have given their circumstances. (Kimberly's mother, Linda Williams, passed away in 2016 after a decade-long battle with early-onset dementia. Kimberly's bestselling memoir, *Where the Light Gets In* [Crown Archetype, 2016] chronicles how Kimberly and her family coped with Linda's illness.)

Another thing I remember from when I was little—and this helps inform what Brad and I are doing now—was the Thanksgiving my parents decided we were going to volunteer at a soup kitchen. I was dolling out turkey and peas in the serving line for hungry people on the other side of the counter, and I remember expecting to see more gratitude. Instead, it was almost the opposite—they seemed resentful. It was something I didn't really understand at the time, but it didn't feel as good as I had hoped it would. Something was missing.

Brad and I have been really inspired by an organization in Santa Barbara called Unity Shoppe. It's basically a food pantry program where enrolled clients can come in once a month and shop for their family. The place is set up like a real grocery store, and people can choose what they want. The woman who started it, Barbara Tellefson, had had similar experiences to mine growing up. She saw people being given handouts that weren't necessarily what they wanted. They didn't have a choice, they were expected to be happy with whatever they got, and consequently they didn't feel the sense of dignity a normal customer might feel when shopping. It wasn't empowering.

We borrowed the ideas we loved from Unity Shoppe and created a nonprofit in Nashville called The Store. The Store community aims to empower and dignify individuals and families who are seeking self-sufficiency by providing choices for healthy food. In this free grocery, we want kids to see their parents making choices for their families. We want to see these families having a normal shopping experience. We also want members of the general community to come and volunteer with their kids.

Brad's dream is to have a little coin-operated horse or merry-go-round out front for kids to ride, because that's what he remembers about going to the grocery store when he was a kid. We've actually gotten a lot of ideas from our own children. Huck and Jasper have come with us to Unity Shoppe to volunteer quite a bit, and they'll be a part of this one too. One of their suggestions is that we provide free samples because that's one of the best things about going to a grocery store. The cheese cubes on toothpicks are their favorite!

BRAD: My first introduction to any kind of charity was when I was a singer as a kid in my hometown in West Virginia. My parents had really good priorities. I'm lucky that way. They weren't interested so much in me becoming famous as a singer. My mom, being a school teacher, and my dad, working for the state highway department, had different perspectives. My mother's main focus as a teacher was, "Well, I don't care what you do musically, but you'd better be a good person." I remember my parents sort of pushing me into singing for people at the local hospital in what they called the "respite ward"—long-term hospice—the area where you had stroke victims, and you had people that needed music, needed something to break up the day. I would go over as a twelve- or thirteen-year-old with a guitar and sing for these people. You can imagine how, as a twelve-year-old kid, I might not look forward to singing at a nursing home or performing for people in a hospital, but I immediately felt the effects of what kindness and good deeds do for your soul.

With our kids, our focus has been on hunger. . . . I remember one year at Thanksgiving, my wife said, "They need to understand, especially this time of the year at Thanksgiving, when the rest of the United States is stuffing its face, that there are people here who don't have enough to eat." The boys were acting a little spoiled and were not happy about having to do something on the start of their holiday break at school, and Kim was really mad at how they were acting. We took them to the Unity Shoppe—it's such a great charity and has become the inspiration for what we're doing in Nashville. I saw my children immediately switch from entitled and spoiled to understanding what was going on in front of their very eyes. They were seeing families there together, and it wasn't a soup kitchen. It was actually a way different concept than that, but it had the same effect as putting food on someone's plate.

Another thing we did early on because of what Kim's mother did with her is Meals on Wheels. Kim would take our youngest, Jasper, and our oldest, Huck, when he was younger, and they would go in the car and drive around Franklin, Tennessee, and drop dinners off for people who couldn't get out.

KIMBERLY: That's the goal: to help people who are in a tough time and struggling to get by. A lot of people at the Unity Shoppe actually have a home; they have a car. It's just they're having trouble making ends meet, and in the interim they need help getting back on their feet.

Ultimately, we'd love to have job training to further help people. The program at the Unity Shoppe is for one year, and I think we'll do something similar to that at The Store in Nashville. At the Unity Shoppe it's something like 80 percent of the people who come for help, after the first year, they never see them again, because it works. It works for a year to help people get back on their feet. It's not meant to be a long-term solution. It's meant to be something to help you in the gap time.

One of the most amazing things I remember from the Unity Shoppe was being there with the kids—they love to scoop the bulk rice and beans, and so they were working doing that, and then they went to work on the cash register to help check people out. I saw this gorgeous woman rolling a cart down the aisle, and she looked up at my kids, and this look of delight came on her face and she said, "Oh, I used to bring my kids here to volunteer."

Now she was one of the recipients. It was a community program, and she had grown up knowing about it and volunteering in it, and then she just came to a point in her life when she needed it. There wasn't shame in that. We're all in this together.

When we were trying to figure out what to call our nonprofit in Nashville, we asked Huck, "How do you think those people feel when they walk through a free grocery store and they're picking food for their family and they go to the checkout line? How do you think they feel?" And he said, "They feel like this," and he made a totally blank face like he was almost bored.

We said, "Well what does that mean?" And he said, "Normal . . . they feel normal."

And we thought, well isn't that something? Because there can be so much anxiety and stress surrounding the idea of food, especially for people who are worried about where their next meal's coming from. And this is something that makes them feel normal. That's why we decided to call it The Store, because we want it to be the most normal experience for them and for their children. And that came from Huck's observation.

Where are you going? We're going to The Store. I love that.

BRAD: When you look at the list of things we need to live, it usually goes oxygen, food, and then shelter. Way down the list, obviously, would be things like a car, a house (because shelter is not the same as a house), and then farther down the list are things like WiFi. It's funny, though, as you go down that list, people will probably skimp on food before they'll skimp on WiFi. It's bizarre to me that priorities can be so out of whack, when you start thinking, "I gotta make this house payment, I gotta make the car payment. What can we do? Well, we could eat cheaper, and I suppose we can skip a meal here and there."

The next thing you know, they're skipping one of the most basic things, and that is, in a nutshell, one of the things that our charity is looking at—people who are down on their luck but haven't hit rock bottom. They're caught between a rock and a hard place and they need food for their family. One of the things a charity needs to do is take away the sting of that moment, and give people dignity. And that can happen as simply as literally saying to your kid, "Come on, we're going to The Store."

KIMBERLY: Ideally at The Store we would teach the people we serve how to garden and have vegetables available so they can become better educated about the dietary needs they have. We would also talk to them about sugar intake. There's so much diabetes in the communities, and, as we know, unfortunately, most of the cheapest food is the worst for you. So, we could offer instruction about basic farming and gardening so they could grow their own and become sustainable on their own.

That's also a way the work here connects with hunger around the world, which is something we want our boys to understand. Through places such as World Vision and ChildFund International, as a family we have "adopted" different kids from different places so that our kids follow their stories. Of course, when we go to places such as Haiti, we come back and tell them about it. Reading books and just learning about the world and sharing stories about what we've seen and showing them pictures and stuff also help connect the dots.

And then just having them do hands-on work helps make the connections even more real. "Look at this whole bucket of beans! Can you imagine that some people don't even have this?" Or, "Look at this clean water. We can just turn on the tap here, and we have it." Just trying to get them to imagine what life is like in other parts of the world helps, so we make it a priority to talk about it, and how it all connects—how women and girls have to go get clean water, and that's why they can't go to school.

Similarly, food and basic nutrition can affect the larger picture of continuing education for a child—to have to work for their family such that they can't go to school, and what that leads to, and how hard it is to break the cycle of poverty when you do that. But I bite my tongue and I try not to say things like, "You need to finish what's on your plate because of starving children in Africa." I know we're not supposed to say that, but I do think it.

Rather than making it a threat or reprimanding them, I think we ought to just start out the meal with grace and gratitude for the food on our table. We try to come at it from a positive angle, and the conversations that I have about it are separate from their own eating or not eating.

Huck loves to say grace. He usually takes the lead on that. When I was little, we always said the same grace: "Bless, oh Lord, this food to our use and our lives to thy love and service and give us thankful hearts through Jesus Christ our Lord. Amen." We said it every day, and I probably didn't know what I was saying. With our family now, we don't use that prayer, but we say a basic prayer of gratitude and thanks and then any special requests, which can go on for a while.

It helps when the boys actually cook the food with me. They're more inclined to eat it, I've found. That's sort of a separate issue, but it's true. I think they have more gratitude when they see where it's coming from and when they actually help make it. (Huck has an affinity for chicken and dumplings.)

We've been getting these Green Chef meals, where they send the ingredients and the recipe. I'm not very creative and I've got like three things I can make, and then everyone gets really bored with them really fast, including myself. So, we'll do Green Chef, and it's fun—the kids will help me with it in the kitchen, it's always different every night, and it has lots of different vegetables, which I like, and it's organic. What I actually *love* about it is we don't throw food away, because if I need two stalks of celery I don't have to buy an entire bunch of celery. They send only the food you're going to use in the recipe. If I have a lot left over, I'll freeze it, or we'll eat it the next day, but I find there's so much less food waste when I use it.

BRAD: You know, there's so much about hunger and poverty in the Bible. And if there's any common theme, it's this philosophy for "the least of these." So it's been very inspiring in Nashville to see that our city, as a sort of people, have adopted a place like Haiti. So many friends of mine, from Carrie Underwood, who is very focused on Haiti, to (the Olympic figure skater) Scott and Tracie Hamilton (who have adopted children from Haiti)—one after another, people I know have discovered Haiti. Having gone there a few times myself, there's nothing like seeing this need for water and food that's just unlike anything I've ever seen. Haiti is, by some estimates, the poorest country in the world—that's extreme.

You don't have to be the poorest country in the world to have hunger problems. I mean, this is one of the wealthiest countries in the world, and we have hunger here too.

For Christians in general, to focus on hunger issues is a great use of their time. The great thing about living in the Bible Belt in Nashville is that there are some really good examples of Christians here. One of my favorite quotes by Mark Twain is, "If Christ were here now, there is one thing he would not be—a Christian."[1] But in Tennessee, I know a lot of examples where that's not the case. I know many people who are living in a way that I think Jesus would give them a thumbs up. There are a lot of ways to get what I would consider to be sidetracked and on the wrong track—getting into things that are not necessarily the point as a Christian.

My point is, if there's anything that boils it down to just the message of Christianity and doing something where you really can't go wrong, it's charity and feeding people who are hungry. What a way to begin a journey as a Christian, you know? In some ways, I wish churches would start there, like, "Oh, you want to be a part of this church? Cool. Come with us because here's what we're doing right now: we're gonna feed people. We're gonna go do that."

You begin a journey with a single step. In terms of making a difference in global hunger, I would imagine the best thing you could do is vote for people who seem to have a heart for helping others. Begin there. And that's in any political party. We're in a moment in time where this partisan thing is happening, but it will pass, and we'll return to more issue-based things.

If there's any way our country can lead in this world, it is by helping people. That's the quickest way to make friends. A friend I worked with in Haiti when we did a lot of work with water systems down there said it's pretty hard to hate the United States when there's a well with an American flag on it pumping water out. That kind of thing is important. While people debate immigration and border security and all of these things—look, you can be on either side of those issues and still believe we need to help feed people in South America.

KIMBERLY: The Store was driven by Brad's passion to do in Tennessee what we'd seen the Unity Shoppe do in California. When we took our kids and saw how much they were getting out of helping and being a part of it and how welcoming Unity Shoppe was to volunteers, he was the one who started saying, "We need to do this everywhere. This needs to happen in Tennessee, and it needs to happen all over the country."

We do need to spread this. It's a great way to give back.

BRAD: What I hope happens with what we're starting is that it does well enough that other places want to do it. I'd love to hear people say, "See how well this is working there? So-and-so maybe wants to start one up here." Because you know they need it in places like Appalachia, for instance. In some ways, that's the closest thing we have to some Third World conditions here in the United States.

If I had to say one last thing about fighting hunger at home and around the world, it would be to seek out the thing that speaks to you and do it. Start somewhere. Take that step.

Editors' Note: At 233 feet below sea level, Bombay Beach, California, is geographically the lowest community in North America with a history of harder-than-hard knocks that can make it feel even lower. Of the three hundred souls who call this salt-dusted town home only about an hour (but a world away) from tony Palm Springs, most live at or below the poverty line. It's a food desert in the middle of the actual desert, and if Miss Aqua's tiny, overpriced convenience store is closed or runs out of milk, it's a nearly one-hundred-mile round trip to the nearest grocery store. The closest gas station is more than twenty miles away, the nearest hospital almost forty miles away, and the town's children (there are a few dozen of school age) must ride the bus two hours each way to get to school. It was once a popular resort on the shores of the Salton Sea before the fresh water became hypersalinated in the 1970s and killed off fish by the millions. Now a skeleton of its former self—a desperately hard place to live perched on the edge of nowhere—Bombay Beach could be the poster child for "forgotten America." There's no public library or WiFi anywhere in town, more than a few residents live without running water or electricity, and in the summer, temperatures regularly climb above 115 degrees Fahrenheit. On the day we visit with Shorty in her home, it's 120.

I used to come here to water-ski when I was a teenager. In 2009, you know how bad the economy was. I actually closed my business—I owned a pet store in San Diego. Well, I had already moved it once, and I just ended up locking the doors November 30 and loading up everything I owned—six dogs, three cats, and a bird—in an RV and moving to the Slabs. (The Slabs, AKA "Slab City," is a community twenty miles south of Bombay Beach where maybe 150 people live, mostly in recreational vehicles or improvised shelters, year-round, driven by poverty or a desire to live "off-the-grid" on massive concrete slabs leftover from abandoned World War II military barracks.)

I started to work for the church up there for about a year, but my partner Bill couldn't handle it out there, so we drove to Bombay one day, and I found this (RV). And it was purple, and I had to have it. I put a down payment on it, which took everything I had left, and made payments on it until it was paid off.

When it comes to hunger, been there, done that. There are still days when I say, well, what are we gonna eat, guys? Food insecurity? I don't know about all that. All I know is if I have two, and you're hungry, I'll give it to you. I think everybody needs to eat. Anybody—ask 'em—if they come to my door, I won't say no. This one screams at me, yells at me, "Stop feeding them! What are you gonna eat?" Don't worry about what I'm gonna eat. Sooner or later, I'll eat. It's just the way I am.

(Shorty's friend AJ comes in to escape the heat. She stays a few blocks away and used to live in a sewer pipe in San Diego. She plops down in one of two easy chairs beneath the window air conditioning unit, finds a box of purple-frosted Pop Tarts, takes one out, and starts eating.)

She knows a lot about hunger too. I was going to send her away, but then I thought, maybe not. AJ, you know a lot about hunger.

("Yeah," AJ says. "I can't remember the last time I had steak and chicken, pork chops, and stuff like that. I just eat noodles.")

Well, God provides. Once in a while I wonder what we're gonna eat, but something comes up. I mean, I've got plenty of beans and rice. I've got probably twenty-five pounds of rice and beans back here. People say, what are you gonna do, feed everybody? And I do.

The nearest *real* grocery store is about fifty miles away. And to get to the market you've gotta pay somebody twenty or thirty bucks just to get there. And then they only want to take you one place, and not stop here and here and here and here. But you're paying all that money and you want to get all your shopping done.

If you buy it here, it will cost you three or four times as much and ends up costing as much as it would have if you'd paid for that ride to the real grocery store.

(Shorty says she tries to get all her shopping for the month done in a single trip. Each Wednesday [except for the second of each month, when she volunteers at a food pantry truck that stops in Bombay Beach] she goes to Mecca, California, about twenty-five miles away, to get a bag of food from Catholic Charities, where she's also been a longtime volunteer in its food programs.)

If the rice and beans ran out, I'd hope it was close to Wednesday and I could go get in line and get more. If that's not an option, I dunno. I have a lot of canned goods. I'd live on fruit because I've got a lot of cans of that in the garage. Canned fruit.

A lot of people have to choose between buying groceries and paying for their medication. I don't take any meds because I don't go to doctors. But if I'm short, my lights are first. Food is second. I don't need that as bad as I need my lights, because I've got to have my air— my dogs will die. Or these guys might need to get out of the streets in the heat. I leave the AC on all the time.

I don't care about me. Either way, God isn't gonna let me go. When I'm done, he'll let me go.

Hunger—it's all over the place, everywhere. And not just in Bombay. Everywhere you go. Look in your big cities where they're laying by the side of the road. Those people are hungry too! It's everywhere. Maybe you look at them and say, yeah, they're hungry because they choose to drink and not eat. Well, you know what? That drink is killing the pain of not being able to eat all the time, so I don't fault them for that.

People need to remember what life is about and help. Because it isn't about how high you can climb and how much money you have when you get there. It's about helping humanity. You're not the only one who has to climb this mountain. Help that guy over there. He needs your help. Don't step on his head so you can get there. Or if you're gonna step on his head, at least give him a hand up afterward.

But it's not your fault, right? You didn't do it. Wait a minute, maybe you did? Ask yourself: Do your actions have any repercussions or connections to why he's out there on the street, hungry?

THE LAMB'S AGENDA

SAMUEL RODRIGUEZ

This is a book about tackling one of the greatest plagues of humanity since the fall: hunger.

We are asking questions such as, How do we respond to the one in nine people on the planet suffering from malnutrition? How should the church respond? And what can we do to lead the charge in combating extreme poverty in developing nations and ending the hunger crisis for families worldwide?

These are big questions, yet the answers are simple.

I have spent my life bearing witness to hunger. Growing up in a Puerto Rican household in Bethlehem, Pennsylvania, I lived in the heart of the Rust Belt, where we watched steel mills shut down, unemployment rise, and homelessness increase during the 1980s and 1990s.

I remember my youth leader calling for us to "feed the hungry" with lessons from Matthew 25, telling us that we should commit our time and energy at homeless shelters, rescue missions, and urban ministries among the newly marginalized.

At the same time, the Central American countries of Guatemala and Nicaragua were in the throes of a civil war. In the aftermath of the communist revolutions, people in both countries were suffering abject poverty and deep hunger.

I traveled to Central America and witnessed the food insecurity of these post-conflict nations firsthand. In Nicaragua, we discovered a three-month-old baby who had been left on the street to die. We found the mother, and when we spoke with her, we asked her why she would abandon her child this way. The answer? She had no food.

As a minister, I am called to preach the gospel of Christ. If I preach it, I must live it as well. Addressing extreme poverty and hunger isn't an option. For Christians, it is as mandatory, inevitable, and real as Jesus feeding the multitudes with just a few loaves and fishes.

We can do this through the miracle of food programs that end malnutrition both here in the United States, in Latin American countries, and across the globe.

Feeding the hungry, providing water for the thirsty, and welcoming the stranger are at the heart of Scripture. They are the quintessential rubric articulated by Jesus Christ himself. From the prophets of the Old Testament who called on the faithful to care for the poor to letters of the apostles in the New Testament—there is a thread that runs through Scripture to care for the marginalized.

Jesus begins his ministry in Luke 4 by quoting Isaiah 61:

The Spirit of the Lord is on me,

> because he has anointed me

> to proclaim good news to the poor.

He has sent me to proclaim freedom for the prisoners

> and recovery of sight for the blind,

to set the oppressed free,

> to proclaim the year of the Lord's favor. (Luke 4:18-19)

No one knew what to say then. Many still do not know what to say.

James tells us, "Religion that God our Father accepts as pure and faultless is this: to look after orphans and widows in their distress and to keep oneself from being polluted by the world" (James 1:27). Indeed it is the very definition of our beliefs and our practice to care for the most vulnerable women and children around the world. And in this case, it means addressing access to proper nutrition.

The cross is a symbol of the vertical and the horizontal. The vertical represents God's eternal, universal truths. The horizontal represents our relationships in the church, society, the market, and even the media. It is the coming together of the left and the right. Orthopraxy and orthodoxy. Justice and righteousness. Sanctification and justification. Compassion and love.

It is the blended messages of the Reverend Dr. Martin Luther King Jr. and the Reverend Billy Graham. It is the united hymns "Just As I Am" and "We Shall Overcome." We are the generation that together can live out the symbolic fullness of the cross. Together.

We don't have an elephant agenda, and we don't have a donkey agenda; we have the Lamb's agenda. This agenda calls us to love, from womb to tomb, and to advocate for the least of these.

Advocacy is the simple practice of offering your voice to uplift those who may be seemingly powerless, voiceless, or hopeless. We are their advocates. We lift up their voices to support full funding for global health and alleviation of poverty, for immigration, pro-life issues, prison reform, and malnutrition. Every life is sacred, made in the image of God.

Jesus is waiting for the church to stand up. Many on the front lines of the pro-life movement forget the calling to support the child born into poverty, hunger, or a life of violence. If we are to live out a truly pro-life ethic for all humans, we must reconsider the critical importance of global nutrition funding to combat hunger and its effects, which often include a lifetime of challenges from physical and cognitive stunting.

Global health issues are also global security interests. In addressing the issues of poverty and health in a low-income nation, we are using "soft power" or "smart power" to tackle larger security problems by building diplomacy and good will among potentially threatening nations. Healthy people mean healthy nations. We must ask ourselves, "What if we do nothing?" I would argue that today's complacency is tomorrow's captivity for the church and for our nation.

Many of us worry about potential governmental corruption, especially abroad. The late Senator Jesse Helms coined the phrase "money down a rat hole," which has been stuck in minds of many conservatives for decades. The answer to the "rat hole" conundrum is to address corruption head-on.

But remember, we are called to poverty alleviation. And ours is a higher calling, no matter the party or politics.

In working with the George W. Bush administration, I had the honor of advising and strategizing about a myriad of issues while promoting our collective commitment to global health and development. We championed the ethic of "compassionate conservatism" and rallied support for his historic and epic President's Emergency Plan for AIDS Relief (PEPFAR) to prevent and treat HIV/AIDS for millions. In 2002, at the height of the HIV/AIDS emergency, fewer than fifty thousand of the nearly twenty-five million people living with HIV/AIDS in sub-Saharan Africa had access to life-saving antiretroviral drugs.

Today, thanks to PEPFAR and President Bush's leadership, more than fourteen million people have access to those miraculous medications. Many argue that it is President Bush's legacy. These are justice issues, and in the tradition of Abraham Lincoln, Bush offered a prophetic voice for the world's poorest and most vulnerable. His leadership to support PEPFAR has saved millions of lives around the globe. It is a powerful example of what we can do with our global health account funding.

Under both the Obama and Trump administrations, we at National Hispanic Christian Leadership Coalition (NHCLC) have supported legislative measures to uplift the poor domestically and internationally. And we have seen tremendous progress. Our nation has led global efforts to cut by half the number of deaths caused by malaria, tuberculosis, and HIV/AIDS; reduce maternal mortality; and increase child survival. All thanks to US leadership—with the church at the helm of the movement.

This is the good news of efficiency and efficacy working hand in hand: unprecedented, historic progress never before seen in the history of humankind—and all with the price tag of less than 1 percent of the entire US budget. A penny to the dollar.

The simple truth is this: as Christians, we are mandated by God, told by the Holy Spirit, and compelled by the Bible to commit ourselves to uplifting the poor and ending avoidable tragedies—including global hunger. We already have borne witness to the elimination of preventable diseases and extreme poverty in the lives of millions.

According to the Lamb's agenda, we are to offer life and life abundantly to those who might otherwise not survive. To those whom much is given, much is expected—and the United States has so very much.

Join us in saving lives through the Christian practice of advocacy on behalf of the marginalized both in the United States and around the world.

TEACH A MAN TO FISH

DIANE BLACK

N early twenty-five years ago, my first journey into the developing world took me to Haiti, the poorest nation in the western hemisphere, with a long history of dictatorship and corruption that has left the country perpetually unstable.

Upon flying into the Caribbean nation, the difference between Haiti and the Dominican Republic—the two countries that share the island of Hispaniola—was stark and immediate. Whereas the Dominican Republic was lush with trees and agriculture, the Haitian side of the island was barren, with erosion contributing to the polluting of streams and bay areas.

When I visited Haiti in the 1990s, Jean-Bertrand Aristide was in power, and prior to his removal by a military coup, he urged his supporters to defeat his opponents by "necklacing"—the brutal practice of placing burning tires around the necks of rivals and their supporters. It was a terrible, dangerous time to live in or even visit the perpetually troubled, impoverished country. Despite the warnings about potential threats to my safety and security, I was determined to go. I traveled with a delegation from the Evangelical Lutheran Church in America (ELCA) who arrived to provide health care and minister to Haitians.

Since that first visit to Haiti, I have traveled all over the world, spending time in Guatemala, Kenya, and other developing nations.

But I have never seen more extreme poverty than what I witnessed in Haiti. I also have rarely seen greater hope amid immense hardship.

The aim of the ELCA contingent, of which I was a member, was twofold: spread the Word of Jesus and his love and help communities combat hunger. What I learned from the Lutherans was the power of teaching good, simple practices for farming, fishing, and managing livestock. The Haitian community that our group served on that trip had no real equipment for deep-water fishing or farming, no animals, and no experience. But instead of only giving the community handouts of rice or other food resources, the ELCA spent time teaching members of the community about the detrimental effects of deforestation and erosion, the basics of gardening, and how to feed and breed animals such as piglets and rabbits so that families could have a consistent and renewable source to fill their bellies.

The Lutherans also brought sewing machines and offered classes in which those interested in becoming tailors and seamstresses learned how to make and sell clothing at their local market—a new and steady income stream for their families and the community at large.

Such methods were successful because the Lutheran visitors listened to their Haitian hosts, analyzed the community's assets, and offered to help build on their existing knowledge and capacity.

As the adage says, "Give a man a fish, and he'll eat for a day. Teach him how to fish, and he'll eat for a lifetime."

●   ●   ●

When it comes to combating extreme poverty, whether in Haiti, Kenya, or Guatemala, I have witnessed time and again the necessity of education in any effort to improve nutrition, hygiene, and the overall quality of life for individual people, families, and whole communities. For example, I recall how in the small bags they carried with them,

Guatemalan mothers often packed containers of water sweetened with sugar for their children. It placated the kids, but it was nothing more than empty calories that promoted tooth decay and cravings for a sugary diet. We spent time explaining the harmful effects of this "sugar water" on their children as a way to change behavior.

As a nurse, I care deeply about providing communities with information about what good nutrition is and how it helps build stronger, healthier brains and bodies. Without proper nutrition, we know mothers suffer from anemia and children suffer from cognitive and physical stunting that limits capabilities throughout their lifespan. Nutrition is the most basic element all humans need to survive.

In recent years, I traveled with a congressional delegation to Kenya to see the amazing advances in health, agriculture, and the economy spurred by US investments. One site we visited contained the most gorgeous rose farm. The community had allocated land not only for agriculture but also for flowers. It turned out that the flowers were among the most beautiful in the world. This rose farm employed many folks in the community, teaching them to produce and market roses, which were shipped internationally.

It was a wonderful story about how ending hunger also can be addressed by teaching the concepts of a market economy and capitalism. In this case, the community established a sustainable industry to combat poverty and hunger through employment, so that workers could buy food and stimulate the economy.

There are many answers to the question of how to end hunger and poverty, but they share a common foundation: self-sufficiency. Cottage industries, such as the ones promoted by the ELCA, provide skills and promote a strong work ethic. We can learn so much from these "small-batch" ministries and nonprofits that understand how best to use an impoverished community's assets to fill in any gaps in education in order to combat extreme poverty most effectively.

Jesus called us to help the poor. He called us to feed the hungry, not only among our neighbors at home—in our case, here in the United States—but also with our neighbors around the world.

This is loving our neighbor—our brothers and sisters in God's family—just as Jesus calls us to do.

ENDING HUNGER STARTS WITH MODERNIZING HOW WE DELIVER FOOD AID

BOB CORKER

W hen I arrived in Uganda in the spring of 2017, Bidi Bidi was the largest refugee camp in the world. My Senate Foreign Relations Committee colleague, Senator Chris Coons (R-DE), and I visited the camp as part of a fact-finding mission to get a firsthand look at one of the world's so-called "four famines"—concurrent disasters in Nigeria, South Sudan, Somalia, and Yemen—that at the time placed an estimated twenty million people in jeopardy.

Our trip reinforced our understanding of the dire need for food assistance and the incredible work of US and international aid organizations in distributing life-saving food to the most vulnerable populations.

Around the world today, seventy-five million people are in danger of starvation, and 800 million people are in need of food aid.

Thanks to the generosity of the American people, the United States is the largest contributor of emergency food aid, much of which is provided through the United Nations World Food Programme. However, we cannot and should not address this challenge alone. In addition to using current resources more efficiently, we must urge other nations to increase their contributions to avert further suffering, violence, and instability.

What we witnessed at Bidi Bidi served as added inspiration for our commitment to modernizing a US international food assistance system that currently prevents our country from getting more food to those in need faster, and all without additional funding.

Existing rules require US sourcing for almost all food aid through the Food for Peace program, half of which must then be shipped on overpriced US-flagged vessels. The program also mandates that 15 percent of all US-donated food first be sold by aid organizations, producing cash that then funds development projects—a practice known as "monetization."

Because of these archaic rules, only 30 cents of every dollar dedicated for this aid pays for food. The rest goes to shipping, handling, and other overhead costs. Making matters worse, shipping food from the United States can take two to five months to reach its intended destination. In the case of the Bidi Bidi camp in Uganda, where refugees nearly filled the camp over the course of weeks, US food aid would have arrived too late, and people would have starved. The US Agency for International Development (USAID) had to use alternative funding exempt from restrictions to purchase food in Uganda, which arrived within weeks and prevented further suffering for refugees.

Tragically, such waste and delays are an issue of life and death. Professor Chris B. Barrett of Cornell University testified before our committee that, for the amount of funding diverted away from food in the Food for Peace program, "We sacrifice roughly forty thousand children's lives annually because of antiquated food aid policies."[1]

Senator Coons and I recently introduced the Food for Peace Modernization Act of 2018 (FPMA) to use our limited food aid resources in the most effective way possible. FPMA would reduce the share of food aid required to be US-sourced from 100 percent to

25 percent, permitting the remaining 75 percent to be procured locally or regionally, including options to provide vouchers and debit cards for individual people to buy food in local markets. This will maximize cost effectiveness.

The legislation would also lift the 15 percent "monetization" requirement. The US Government Accountability Office has warned this process is "inefficient and can cause adverse market impacts" in recipient countries.[2] Taken together, these reforms could free up as much as $275 million, which could then be used to more quickly feed nearly nine million more people.

Modernizing our food aid programs does not mean eliminating US commodities in the system, since local and regional markets cannot provide enough food to cover all the disasters around the globe. These changes would put all options on the table, providing USAID the flexibility to choose the right type of food aid for each situation. At no extra taxpayer expense, we can put more food into food aid and have it arrive months faster to feed millions of additional starving people without reducing the critical role of American farmers.

We have made substantial progress in recent years building support among stakeholders for these reforms, including from the American Farm Bureau Federation. The 2018 Farm Bill currently being considered in Congress provides the opportunity to more fully modernize our food aid efforts when there is enormous need around the world, and I am hopeful with bipartisan support in both the House and Senate that we will ultimately be successful.

Our long-term objective is to build resiliency from food crises through sustainable development. But at a time of unprecedented shortages facing so many people around the world and budget deficits at home, the United States first needs to use every dollar more efficiently to save more lives today.

EXODUS FROM HUNGER

DAVID BECKMANN

My first job was in a little village in northwest Bangladesh, and it was a joy to return to the same village many years later. I was struck by the dramatic progress my old friends—and Bangladesh as a whole—have made in recent decades. Women have more freedom than they did, children are visibly better nourished, and more foods are available in the markets.

On my return visit, I reconnected with Mr. Bari, who taught at the village school. He had a thatch house then; now it's cinder block with a tin roof. The gulley next to his house, where mosquitoes used to breed, has been filled. The village used to be isolated, especially in the rainy season, but today buses run up and down an asphalt road to town. Mr. Bari said he thanks almighty God that his life has turned out so much better than he expected.

Bangladesh and many other developing countries have made dramatic progress against hunger, poverty, and disease. In 1990, two billion of the world's people were caught in extreme poverty. In the intervening not-quite thirty years, that number has dropped to about 750 million.

Progress against hunger and poverty in the United States has not been as dramatic, but we also have made progress in recent decades. A team of prominent physicians who visited poor US communities in the 1960s found children with bloated bellies.[1] The government antipoverty programs that began with presidents Lyndon Johnson and Richard Nixon have substantially reduced hunger and poverty. Without them, the US poverty rate would be almost double what it is today.[2]

For people who believe in God, the escape by hundreds of millions of people from hunger is cause for praise and thanksgiving. This is an experience of our loving God among us—like the biblical exodus. And God is inviting all of us to help continue the progress that so clearly is possible.

Based on progress in recent years, all the governments of the world agreed in 2016 on ambitious global goals for 2030 called the Sustainable Development Goals. Among them is the goal of ending hunger worldwide by 2030. There would still be pockets of hunger— groups of people with special problems (addiction, for example) and countries suffering from war or tyranny. But if we could tilt the global trend line upwards just a bit, we would virtually end hunger within a decade or two.

We have no guarantee that we successfully can end hunger by 2030. In fact, we have suffered serious setbacks since the global goals were adopted. The forces in US politics that want to cut back on focused efforts to reduce poverty have gained strength. At the same time, violence and climate change have led to more severe hunger in some countries.

Yet we have biblical promises that God is working for good in the world and is especially concerned about people in need. The passage that I find particularly meaningful in coping with recent setbacks comes from Psalm 31:24: "Be strong and take heart, /all you who hope in the Lord."

HELP FROM SCIENCE

I remember reading an article from the January 2008 issue of the British medical journal *Lancet* about how the Bill & Melinda Gates

Foundation and the World Bank had financed evaluations of various efforts around the world to reduce child malnutrition. The article summarized what these scientific studies had concluded, and demonstrated the severity of the damage malnutrition does to infants and young children—most notably, the permanent damage it often does to a child's brain. It also presented a list of the most cost-effective ways to reduce child malnutrition.

I jumped out of my chair and went running to the office of a colleague, Asma Lateef, director of the Bread for the World Institute. We had both spent many years working on various strategies to reduce child hunger. But now that one article gave us evidence-based conclusions about the strategies that have the biggest impact. For instance, most nutrition programs in the world are not focused on pregnant women and children younger than the age of two. Many parents in poverty don't know that breastfeeding is better than infant formula, and that hand-washing with soap prevents dysentery and diarrhea. The top-line finding was that limited dollars should be focused on pregnant women and children up to the age of two—the first one thousand days of life.

The Bill & Melinda Gates Foundation and the World Bank convened key organizations from around the world that work on child hunger, urging us to reshape our efforts based on the new evidence. The action program that emerged from those discussions was called Scaling Up Nutrition.

By coincidence or providence, this new knowledge became available just before a global jump in grain prices provoked a surge in hunger around the world. The Bush administration increased food aid right away. The Obama administration came to power at the beginning of 2009 with the powerful idea of leading an international campaign to help poor farmers in poor countries increase their agricultural production.

President Barack Obama committed more than $1 billion per year in increased US aid for food security. Bread for the World and our members across the nation helped convince Congress to approve the US funding. With leadership from the US government, other governments committed more than ten times that amount. And local efforts more than matched international assistance.

The US global food security initiative was named Feed the Future. US Secretary of State Hillary Rodham Clinton's staff met repeatedly with nongovernmental organizations, including Bread for the World. We urged the administration to include the newly available, evidence-based nutrition action plan in their strategy. We also urged Congress to provide funding specifically for nutrition.

Bread for the World's network of concerned people and churches weighed in—eighteen organizations of Christian women mounted campaigns, and five thousand women petitioned Secretary Clinton directly. Twenty-five women even made scrapbooks about the importance of nutrition in the first one thousand days in a child's life and presented these scrapbooks to their members of Congress.

Happily, Secretary Clinton decided to promote Scaling Up Nutrition, which she gave a catchier name: 1,000 Days. It became part of Feed the Future. Between 2011 and 2018, US support for work with small-scale farm families in nineteen countries brought twenty-three million people out of extreme poverty, and nutrition assistance to those families spared three million young children from stunting.[3] We have seen that child stunting can be reduced more quickly than we thought possible. The number of stunted children in the world (zero to five years old) has dropped by fifteen million in five years (2012–2017).[4]

POLITICAL WILL IS THE BINDING CONSTRAINT

The binding constraint on progress against hunger is the lack of sufficient political will. While the US government and other governments globally are contributing substantially to progress against hunger, they could and should do more. It is the single most important factor in making progress against hunger that is possible and that our loving God surely desires.

Churches and charities provide important assistance to hungry people. Businesses organize employment opportunities, and the best way for a family to escape hunger is a good job. Yet government policies and programs are crucial to achieving progress against hunger, and political leaders—and voters—typically have other priorities.

President Donald Trump and our present Congress both have proposed budgets that would cut funding for US programs that help low-income Americans by more than $2 trillion over the next decade. If US churches wanted to try to make up for such proposed cuts in assistance, every church in the country would have to raise and give away an additional $700,000 each year for the next ten years! Anybody who is active in a church knows it would be impossible.

President Trump also has proposed cutting international aid especially deeply—by one-third. US food assistance is keeping millions of refugees and other people from starving, and yet President Trump has proposed even deeper cuts in humanitarian food assistance.

Bread for the World and an array of other faith-based groups have opposed all these funding cuts—with remarkable success. We advocate for reforms that make government programs more effective, but we don't think our country is spending too much money to help hungry and poor people. We are concerned about the federal deficit, but almost none of the recent surge in deficit spending has gone to people in poverty. In fact, international aid amounts to only 1 percent of federal spending.

Thankfully, when specific cuts have come up for consideration, some Republicans have joined Democrats in opposing them. A bipartisan group of members of Congress staunchly has opposed President Trump's proposed cuts to international aid. Bread for the World and its members have helped win additional aid to four countries in North Africa and the Middle East (northern Nigeria, South Sudan, Somalia, and Yemen) that are facing famine.

GOD'S CALL TO CHRISTIANS

Bread for the World is a Christian advocacy movement to end hunger. Our network includes 2.5 million people, five thousand local churches, a growing web of partner organizations, and about five thousand deeply committed volunteer leaders. We work in a bipartisan way, and we have long-standing partnerships with a wide array of church bodies—Catholic and Protestant, conservative and liberal, and racially diverse. Bread for the World and its members have a long record of advocacy achievements, and the key to these achievements is the advocacy of committed Christians across the country.

Based on the proven effectiveness of Feed the Future and 1,000 Days, both parties in Congress joined together in 2016 to pass the Global Food Security Act. No one knew at the time who would win the presidential election that year, but the Global Food Security Act mandated that the next administration continue our country's effective programs of agriculture and nutrition assistance. Individual people and churches in Bread for the World worked with the networks of partner organizations to build support for this legislation.

For example, Rev. Ron Neustadt in Belleville, Illinois, called his member of Congress, US Representative Mike Bost. Ron managed to speak to the congressman's legislative director, who had not yet heard about the Global Food Security Act. When a week passed, and Ron hadn't heard back, he called again. Several of his friends also called. Congressman Bost decided to cosponsor the bill. In all, 127 members of the House cosponsored.

An impressive list of cosponsors helped to convince congressional leadership to bring the bill up for a vote, and it passed with big bipartisan majorities in both houses. In 2018, Congress reauthorized the Global Security Act for another five years. Bread for the World and our partners urged the US President and Congress to further expand US nutrition assistance and lead the world in a campaign to overcome child malnutrition.

It is not an accident that Christian groups provide an essential constituency for programs that help hungry people in our country and worldwide. Sociological studies have confirmed that people who experience God as a loving presence in their lives are more inclined to support government policies and programs that help people in need.[5] Christians experience the love and mercy of God in Jesus Christ. The embrace of God moves Christians to share God's love with other people, especially people in need. "Dear friends, since God so loved us, we also ought to love one another" (1 John 4:11).

God invites us to work for changes that will make the world more consistent with God's love for everyone. Our loving God has made it possible to end hunger in our generation—and is inviting us, US Christians, to contribute to this great exodus from hunger.

ACKNOWLEDGMENTS

Jenny Dyer would like to offer deep gratitude to the Eleanor Crook Foundation's executive director, Will Moore, for his vision and support to create this book. We appreciate your trust in us to craft this unique compilation of essays that we hope will play a role in ushering in the end of hunger during our lifetime.

Special thanks to Senator-Doctor Bill Frist for his leadership and mentorship at Hope Through Healing Hands. His experience, passion, and leadership in the global health arena has been a beacon for all working to end extreme poverty and disease around the world.

Many thanks to the Hope Through Healing Hands team, Jen St. Clair, Amy Fogleman, and Jane Lynch Crain, who provided immense support by organizing, managing, and editing this book.

Thank you to everyone at InterVarsity Press for believing in this important project.

Finally, with much appreciation and love to my husband, John, and my two sons, Rhys and Oliver.

Cathleen Falsani would like to thank her husband, Maurice, and son, Vasco, for their support, patience, and collaboration during the creation of this important book.

To Casey Cora, a prince among men by any measure: my deep thanks for your help with this project and for being such an extraordinarily loving member of our tribe.

A special word of thanks to B, Gayle, Jamie, Rudo, Roxy, Tom, Abby, and all my friends, mentors, and coconspirators at the ONE Campaign for your persistence, resistance, and insistence in working on behalf of the world's poor.

Thank you to Botherjohn Spoon, Theresa Lamer, and AJ in Bombay Beach; to Dave Day, Pastor Saul Solano Guzman, and Esther Genaro Pacheco from Growers First; and a special gracias, querida, to Carolyn Reyes for mobile translation and transcription services (rendered at thirty-five thousand feet and on deadline).

Dhanyavad to Rupa, David, and Gautham Rai, and the whole Rai family in Kathmandu.

A deep bow of gratitude to Ethan McCarthy, Cindy Bunch, Helen Lee, Andrew Bronson, and the entire crew at InterVarsity Press for their full-throated, unequivocal support for this project from the moment we introduced it to them. And to Sally Sampson Craft—I'm so glad we ran into each other at the airport. Thank you for taking the project to your wonderful IVP colleagues.

Once more with feeling, to my many generous friends who answered the call when they got it and donated their time, effort, words, and stories to this book—you amaze me, and we could not have done this without you. Thank you. Zikomo kwambiri.

And to Linda Richardson, for giving me wings all those years ago.

NEXT STEPS

Advocacy and Philanthropy

O ur goal for this book has been to both educate and activate. We hope to have informed you well with some of the leading experts on hunger, famine, and nutrition, and in turn, we are optimistic you are ready to do something, get involved, and join the campaign to end hunger. For Christians and people of faith, the first thing we recommend is consideration of participation through prayer and meditation. We find that this quiet reflection gives clarity and wisdom for each person to find how God might be leading them to use their special gifts, talents, and skill sets to affect some of the world's greatest challenges.

Secondly, we invite you to donate. We welcome your time and your resources. There are wonderful nonprofit organizations tackling hunger on the front lines of poverty, both in the United States and around the world. Please see the following short list of those with whom we work and with whom we recommend you consider getting involved.

Finally, and perhaps most importantly, we welcome you to advocate on behalf of those living with hunger. You've read the book. You've heard the stories. We know what makes a difference and how to make a difference, but we need your voice. Every single person has the power to affect the lives of millions. Advocacy is going upstream to tackle the roots of the problem, through funding infrastructure and systems designed to address hunger in smart, efficient, and scientific ways, for instance, during the first one thousand days of a child's life.

ADVOCACY

How do you advocate?

How do you take that first step to raise your voice to combat hunger? It's simple, and it's easy.

Our ask is that you go to senate.gov or house.gov and simply research your members of Congress by inputting your zip code to find their offices and emails. Next, consider calling, emailing, or even tweeting your member of Congress with the following letter:

Dear President/Senator/Representative _____,

As a constituent, I write to urge you to protect and increase funding for US programs for global nutrition.

As a person of faith, I care deeply about the health of vulnerable populations worldwide. Currently, one in three persons suffers from malnutrition, which has devastating consequences particularly for mothers and children in the first one thousand days of life. Cognitive and physical stunting and wasting are a lifetime tragedy leading to chronic disease, an impaired immune system, and inhibited intellectual development for individuals. Malnutrition is the root of nearly half of under-five child deaths globally each year (approximately three million deaths).

The good news is that we can change that. We know that proper interventions during pregnancy, including foods rich in folic acid, iron, and vitamin A, can alter the course of a child's life. With the prevention of anemia in the mother and encouragement of breastfeeding for the first year of life for the child, lives can be offered a full potential for healthy growth and flourishing.

Unfortunately, the US government and our donor partners commit less than one percent of our foreign assistance funding to programs that specifically focus on combating malnutrition. It is time to reconsider this approach and to make new, bold investments to combat global malnutrition in order to achieve a safer, healthier world for all.

Thank you for your service. We are counting on your leadership and support for healthier families around the world.

Sincerely,

name _____

title _____

city, state _____

PHILANTHROPY

1,000 Days Campaign—1,000 Days Campaign is the leading nonprofit organization working in the United States and around the world to improve nutrition and ensure women and children have the healthiest first one thousand days.

thousanddays.org

Alliance to End Hunger—Alliance to End Hunger engages diverse institutions to build the public and political will to end hunger at home and abroad.

alliancetoendhunger.org

Bread for the World—Bread for the World is a collective Christian voice urging our nation's decision makers to end hunger at home and abroad.

bread.org

CARE—CARE works around the globe to save lives, defeat poverty, and achieve social justice.

care.org

Catholic Relief Services (CRS)—CRS works with organizations around the world to help poor and vulnerable people overcome emergencies, earn a living through agriculture, and access affordable health care.

crs.org

Compassion International—Compassion International exists as a Christian child advocacy ministry that releases children from spiritual, economic, social, and physical poverty and enables them to become responsible, fulfilled Christian adults.

compassion.com

The Eleanor Crook Foundation (ECF)—ECF is a growing US philanthropy committed to research, capacity building, and advocacy to end global malnutrition.

eleanorcrookfoundation.org

Feed the Hungry—Feed the Hungry is dedicated to feeding the poor and hungry around the world, empowering the church worldwide, and sharing the hope that comes through Jesus Christ.

feedthehungry.org

Hope Through Healing Hands (HTHH)—HTHH is a humanitarian organization dedicated to improving the quality of life for citizens and communities around the world.

hopethroughhealinghands.org

Save the Children—Save the Children is the world's top independent charity for children in need. They save children's lives and help them reach their full potential.

savethechildren.org

Share Our Strength—Share Our Strength's mission is to end hunger and poverty in the United States and abroad.

shareourstrength.org

Texas Hunger Initiative (THI)—THI is a capacity building, collaborative project dedicated to developing and implementing strategies to end hunger through policy, education, research, community organizing, and community development.

baylor.edu/texashunger

The ONE Campaign—ONE is a campaigning and advocacy organization of more than nine million people around the world taking action to end extreme poverty and preventable disease, particularly in Africa.

one.org

UN World Food Programme (WFP)—The WFP is the leading humanitarian organization saving lives and changing lives, delivering food assistance in emergencies and working with communities to improve nutrition and build resilience.

wfp.org

World Vision—World Vision is a Christian humanitarian organization dedicated to working with children, families, and their communities worldwide to reach their full potential by tackling the causes of poverty and injustice.

worldvision.org

GLOSSARY

anemia

Anemia is a condition in which the number and size of red blood cells is so low, it impairs the ability of the blood to transport oxygen around the body. The result is an overall decline in health, including loss of energy and reduced physical capacity. In particular, maternal anemia is associated with illness and death of both the mother and baby, including increased risk of miscarriages, stillbirths, premature birth, and low birth weight.

antiretroviral therapy (ARVs)

The human immunodeficiency virus (HIV) is a type of virus called a retrovirus, and the drugs that are used to treat it are called antiretrovirals (ARVs). When a number of ARVs are combined to treat an HIV-positive patient, it's known as antiretroviral therapy (ART). While a cure for HIV does not exist yet at time of publication, if taken correctly, ART can keep a person who is HIV-positive alive for many years while reducing the chance of transmitting the disease to another person. ART reduces the amount of virus (or viral load) in a patient's blood and bodily fluids. ART has been around in various forms since the 1990s, and it is responsible for the precipitous decline in HIV/AIDS-related deaths since the turn of the past millennium. ART is recommended for all people living with HIV, regardless of how long they've had the virus or how healthy they are.

Community-Based Organizations (CBOs)

CBOs are typically implementing organizations in country, on the ground, who are on the front lines of combating a problem or crisis, such as hunger and malnutrition.

Eucharist

Also called the Last Supper or the Lord's Table, among other names, Eucharist is the Christian sacrament or ritual that commemorates the meal Jesus had with his disciples the night before he was crucified. It is part of the Catholic mass and other Christian liturgies.

famine

Famine is a widespread scarcity of food, caused by several human-made factors, including war, inflation, crop failure, population imbalance, or government policies. This phenomenon is usually accompanied or followed by regional malnutrition, starvation, epidemic, and increased mortality.

Farm Bill

The Farm Bill was once dominated by farm support programs, yet it has evolved into an enormous omnibus bill that addresses a wide range of issues, spanning nutrition assistance, rural development, international food aid, and more. This bill influences the food we eat, how it's grown, and the lives of the farmers who grow it. Funding for agricultural research and development only makes up a tiny sliver of the Farm Bill's budget—about 0.2 percent in the 2014 bill—but it has profound consequences for US agricultural competitiveness and global food security.

fasting

Fasting is the practice of abstaining from, or reduction in intake of, food and/or liquids for a period of time. Various religious traditions worldwide practice fasting, often coupled with prayer and meditation.

Feed the Future (FtF)

FtF is the US government's global hunger and food security initiative to give families and communities in some of the world's poorest countries the freedom and opportunity to lift themselves out of food insecurity and malnutrition. This program helps to improve agricultural production and markets and create new opportunities for security and prosperity; strengthen the resilience of communities to shocks that can lead to famine and political unrest; reduce hunger and improve nutrition, especially among mothers and children; and increase the exchange of ideas, technologies, and products that benefit citizens at home and communities abroad.

first one thousand days

The first one thousand days is the period between conception and a child's second birthday. It is the window in which nutrition for the mother and the child is paramount to combat anemia, stunting, wasting, and chronic malnutrition. These have lifelong effects on the child such as chronic illness, lowered ability for learning or reaching educational goals, and a lifetime of lost earning potential.

Food for Peace

This program provides US food aid for emergencies and funds long-term development programs that support nutrition and build resilience.

Food for Peace Modernization Act 2018 (FPMA)

This bill hopes to improve the effectiveness of US food aid. Its proposed reforms include providing USAID the authority to use tools such as vouchers, electronic transfers, and local food purchases, eliminating the requirement to monetize food aid, and reducing the US purchased commodities preference to 25 percent of the Food for Peace budget. It is estimated that the savings from these measures could help feed nine million more people.

food insecurity

Food insecurity is "a household-level economic and social condition of limited or uncertain access to adequate food."[1] It can also simply mean "struggling to avoid hunger," "hungry, or at risk of hunger," and "hungry, or faced by the threat of hunger."

foreign aid

Foreign aid or assistance includes governmental funding, food, and other resources given to other countries in need.

Global Food Security Act (GFSA)

The GFSA in 2016 reduced hunger across the world by investing in the agricultural practices of developing nations. Some methods used to fight hunger included increased attention on agricultural growth, increased farmer productivity, and improved food quality for women and children specifically. This act can help provide healthy food to those in impoverished countries, spur sustainable economic growth in those countries, and improve US national security. The reauthorization of this act in 2018 extends it until 2023.

Global Fund for HIV/AIDS, Tuberculosis, and Malaria (GFATM)

The GFATM is a multilateral organization in which the United States is a key investor. US legislation dictates that for every $1 we contribute to this fund, other nations must contribute $2. This funding goes to implementers in more than 135 nations worldwide to provide prevention and treatment for HIV/AIDS, tuberculosis, and malaria. To date, it is estimated that more than twenty-two million lives have been saved because of this fund.

HIV/AIDS

The human immunodeficiency virus (HIV) is a type of virus called a retrovirus. It harms one's immune system by destroying the white blood cells that fight infection, putting one at risk for serious infections and certain cancers. AIDS stands for acquired immunodeficiency syndrome. It is the final stage of infection with HIV. Not everyone with HIV develops AIDS.

hunger

Hunger is a condition in which a person, for a sustained period, is unable to eat sufficient food to meet basic nutritional needs.

immigrants

Persons who come to live permanently in a foreign country.

infant mortality

Infant mortality is the death of young children under the age of one. This death toll is measured by the infant mortality rate (IMR), which is the number of deaths of children under one year of age per one thousand live births.

malnutrition

Malnutrition refers to the excess, deficit, or imbalances in a person's intake of energy and/or nutrients. This can refer to both under-nutrition and a lack of micronutrients, or it can refer to being over-weight or obese. Currently, one out of three people in the world suffers from malnutrition of some form.

maternal mortality

Maternal mortality is attributed to complications during pregnancy, childbirth, or postpartum. Hemorrhaging is the most common cause of mortality for mothers. Eighty percent of all maternal deaths are preventable.

migrants

Persons who are living and working outside their country of origin.

Non-Governmental Organizations (NGOs)

NGOs are typically nonprofit organizations which may be implementing organizations that are active in humanitarian, educational, health care, public policy, social, human rights, environmental, and other areas to affect changes according to their objectives.

obesity

Obesity affects an estimated forty-one million children worldwide. Children who are overweight or obese, at BMI of 30 or higher, are at a higher risk of developing serious health problems, including type 2 diabetes, high blood pressure, asthma and other respiratory problems, sleep disorders, and liver disease. They may also suffer from psychological effects, such as low self-esteem, depression, and social isolation. Children who are obese are also at risk for noncommunicable diseases, premature death, and disability in adulthood.

President's Emergency Plan for AIDS Relief (PEPFAR)

President George W. Bush launched PEPFAR in 2003 with historic funding for the prevention, care, and treatment of HIV/AIDS. It also supports children affected and infected by HIV/AIDS.

President's Malaria Initiative (PMI)

President George W. Bush launched PMI in 2005 with funding to treat, prevent, and control malaria with the vision of ending preventable child and maternal deaths. This program also builds government capacity to treat and prevent malaria.

Reach Every Mother and Child Act (REACH)

A bill to implement policies, expand proven solutions, and build infrastructure to end preventable maternal, newborn, and child deaths globally.

refugees

Persons who have been forced to flee their country because of persecution, war, or violence.

stunting

Stunting refers to the results of chronic malnutrition on a child, which causes low height for one's age. It can also refer to cognitive stunting, the impairment and underdevelopment of the brain in children due to chronic malnutrition. Stunting is irreversible and can continue after birth as a result of poor feeding practices, repeated infections, and diets that do not give young children the nutrition they need to grow and develop properly.

Sub-Saharan Africa

Sub-Saharan Africa is the area of the African continent that lies south of the Sahara Desert.

Sustainable Development Goals (SDGs)

SDGs are set forth by the United Nations as the blueprint to achieve a better and more sustainable future for all. They address the global challenges we face, including those related to poverty, inequality, climate, environmental degradation, prosperity, peace, and justice. The Goals interconnect and share the target date of 2030.

US Agency for International Development (USAID)

USAID is an independent agency of the US government and leads international development and humanitarian efforts to save lives, reduce poverty, strengthen democratic governance, and help people progress beyond assistance. It is supported by US funding for global health and development

US Foreign Assistance Programs

US Foreign Assistance Programs, or the International Affairs Account, constitutes only one percent of the US federal budget. This Account includes both global health funding (HIV/AIDS, TB, Malaria, International Family Planning, Nutrition, Maternal and Child Health) as well as development funding (education, agriculture, clean water, vaccines) among other services for those living in developing nations.

undernutrition

Undernutrition, or undernourishment, is simply not getting enough calories, protein, or micronutrients as needed for recommended age development.

wasting

Wasting, or low weight for height, is a strong predictor of mortality among children under five. It is usually the result of acute significant food shortage or disease.

World Health Organization (WHO)

The World Health Organization is a specialized agency of the United Nations that is concerned with international public health. Its primary role is to direct international health within the United Nations' system and to lead partners in global health responses.

NOTES

INTRODUCTION

[1] Those living in extreme poverty here are defined as living at $1.25 per day, the decrease was from 36 percent of the world's population to 15 percent of the population. United Nations (UN), "The Millennium Development Goals Report 2015," www.un.org/millenniumgoals/2015_MDG_Report /pdf/MDG%202015%20rev%20(July%201).pdf.

[2] "Sustainable Development Goals," United Nations, accessed March 26, 2019, www.un.org/sustainabledevelopment/sustainable-development -goals.

2. THE END OF HUNGER (JEFFREY D. SACHS)

[1] World Bank, *Taking on Inequality: Poverty and Shared Prosperity 2016* (Washington, DC: World Bank, 2016), https://openknowledge.worldbank .org/bitstream/handle/10986/25078/9781464809583.pdf.

[2] "Obesity and Overweight," World Health Organization, February 16, 2018, www.who.int/news-room/fact-sheets/detail/obesity-and -overweight.

[3] "GDP, Current Prices," International Monetary Fund, accessed March 26, 2019, www.imf.org/external/datamapper/NGDPD@WEO/OEMDC /ADVEC/WEOWORLD.

[4] "Development Aid Stable in 2017 with More Sent to Poorest Countries," The Organisation for Economic Co-operation and Development, April 9, 2018, www.oecd.org/dac/financing-sustainable-development /development-finance-data/ODA-2017-detailed-summary.pdf.

[5] "Billionaires: The Richest People in the World," *Forbes*, March 5, 2019, www .forbes.com/billionaires/#3af20b6a251c.

[6] US Department of Health and Human Services, *Health, United States, 2016: With Chartbook on Long-term Trends in Health* (Hyattsville, MD: National Center for Health Statistics, 2016), www.cdc.gov/nchs/data/hus/hus16 .pdf#053.

[7] See Robert H. Lustig, *The Hacking of the American Mind: The Science Behind the Corporate Takeover of Our Bodies and Brains* (New York: Avery, 2017).

[8] Arielle Duhaime-Ross, "New US Food Guidelines Show the Power of Lobbying, not Science," The Verge, January 7, 2016, www.theverge.com /2016/1/7/10726606/2015-us-dietary-guidelines-meat-and-soda-lobbying -power.

[9] "Sustainable Development Goals," United Nations, accessed March 26, 2019, www.un.org/sustainabledevelopment/sustainable-development -goals.

[10] "Sustainable Development Goals."

[11] Hansen, et al., "Young People's Burden: Requirement of Negative CO_2 emissions," Earth Systems Dynamics 8 (2017): 577, www.earth-syst-dynam .net/8/577/2017/esd-8-577-2017.pdf.

3. A THREAT TO HEALTH ANYWHERE IS A THREAT TO PEACE EVERYWHERE (WILLIAM H. FRIST)

[1] Crystal Lam, "2018 World Hunger and Poverty Facts and Statistics," Hunger Notes, May 25, 2018, www.worldhunger.org/world-hunger-and -poverty-facts-and-statistics/.

[2] "Prevalence of Stunting Among Children Under 5 Years of Age," World Health Organization, updated April 16, 2018, http://apps.who.int/gho /data/node.xgswcah.25.

[3] "The State of Food Security and Nutrition in the World," Food and Agriculture Organization of the United Nations, accessed March 20, 2019, www.fao.org/state-of-food-security-nutrition/en.

[4] Louisiana Lush, Ernest Darkoh, and Segolame L. Ramotlhwa, "Botswana," in The HIV Pandemic, edited by Eduard J. Beck, Nicholas Mays, Alan W. Whiteside, Jose M. Zuniga (Oxford: Oxford University Press, 2006), 181; "Life Expectancy at Birth, Total (Years)," The World Bank, accessed March 20, 2019, https://data.worldbank.org/indicator/SP.DYN.LE00 .IN?locations=ZG.

[5] US President's Emergency Plan for AIDS Relief, "PEPFAR Latest Global Results," November 1, 2018, www.pepfar.gov/documents/organization /287811.pdf; "Global Statistics," HIV.gov, accessed March 20, 2019, www.hiv .gov/hiv-basics/overview/data-and-trends/global-statistics.

[6] Deborah Birx, "World AIDS Day 2018—PEPFAR Reauthorized and 17 Million Lives Saved," DIPNOTE, November 30, 2018, https://blogs .state.gov/stories/2018/11/30/en/world-aids-day-2018-pepfar-reauthorized -and-17-million-lives-saved.

[7]"WFP Says Hunger Kills More Than AIDS, Malaria, Tuberculosis Combined," World Food Programme, June 4, 2009, www.wfp.org/content /wfp-says-hunger-kills-more-aids-malaria-tuberculosis-combined.

[8]M. Shekar, et al., "Investing In Nutrition: The Foundation for Development. An Investment Framework to Reach the Global Nutrition Targets," The World Bank, 2016, http://documents.worldbank.org/curated/en /963161467989517289/pdf/104865-REVISED-Investing-in-Nutrition -FINAL.pdf.

4. THE BIBLE, POVERTY, JUSTICE, AND CHRISTIAN OBEDIENCE (RON SIDER)

[1]When I collected them all in a book, it took about two hundred pages: *Cry Justice: The Bible Speaks on Hunger and Poverty* (Downers Grove: Inter-Varsity Press, 1980); rev. ed., *For They Shall Be Fed* (Dallas: Word Publishing, 1997).

[2]I have written at length on these topics in my *Rich Christians in an Age of Hunger*, 6th ed. (Nashville: Nelson, 2015) and *Just Politics* (Grand Rapids: Baker, 2012).

[3]For further discussion of the concept of social sin and unjust societal systems in both Testaments, see my *Rich Christians in an Age of Hunger*, 115-26.

[4]Chapters 8 and 11 of my *Rich Christians in an Age of Hunger* deal at length with these issues.

[5]For a more lengthy treatment of this topic, see my *Just Politics*, 77-99.

[6]Whether texts accurately describe historical developments or not, they nonetheless reflect the social ideal of the biblical canon.

[7]Both Testaments also teach that society should provide a generous sufficiency for people (young, old, disabled) who cannot care for themselves. See my *Just Politics*, 96-98.

[8]See my detailed discussion of these topics in chapters 8 and 11 in my *Rich Christians in an Age of Hunger*.

5. A MULTIPRONGED APPROACH (RUDO KWARAMBA-KAYOMBO)

[1]FEWSNET (Famine Early Warning Systems Network) and other early warning and early action systems are now in place to help government and humanitarian actors to know in advance what weather patterns they can

expect to hit their countries or areas of operation. Armed with this early warning information countries and humanitarian actors are informed in time to prepare—but we see continuing failure to act on time. Swaziland in 2015–2016 is a case in point.

[2]According to a statement by the public works minister at the time, Saviour Kasukuwere, quoted in "Zimbabwe Declares 'State of Disaster' Due to Drought," *The Guardian*, February 5, 2016, www.theguardian.com/world /2016/feb/05/zimbabwe-declares-state-of-disaster-drought-robert -mugabe.

6. ONWARD TO 2030 (WILL MOORE)

[1]Jennifer E. Dyer and Brian L. Heuser, "How U.S. Conservatives Perceive and Respond to International Nutrition Issues, and How to Shape Messaging for Successful Advocacy," *Christian Journal for Global Health* 5, no. 1 (July 2018): 32-33, https://doi.org/10.15566/cjgh.v5i1.207.

[2]"Children: Reducing Mortality," World Health Organization, September 19, 2018, www.who.int/news-room/fact-sheets/detail/children-reducing -mortality.

[3]Max Roser, "Child Mortality," Our World in Data, https://ourworldindata .org/child-mortality. Accessed March 19, 2019.

[4]World Bank, "Ending Extreme Poverty: Progress, but Uneven and Slowing," *Piecing Together the Poverty Puzzle: Poverty and Shared Prosperity 2018*, https://openknowledge.worldbank.org/bitstream/handle/10986 /30418/9781464813306.pdf.

[5]"The Expert Panel Findings," The Copenhagen Consensus, accessed March 20, 2019, www.copenhagenconsensus.com/copenhagen-consensus -iii/outcome.

7. A PATH TO PEACE AND STABILITY (DAVID BEASLEY)

[1]Food and Agriculture Organization of the United Nations, *The State of Food Security and Nutrition in the World 2018: Building Climate Resilience for Food Security and Nutrition* (Rome, Italy: FAO, 2018), www.fao.org/3 /I9553EN/i9553en.pdf.

[2]"Global Report on Food Crises 2018" Food Security Information Network, 2018, https://docs.wfp.org/api/documents/WFP-0000069227 /download/?_ga=2.67966353.1070572661.1546420321-237976106.15329588 98, 2.

[3]Food and Agriculture Organization of the United Nations, *The State of Food Security and Nutrition in the World 2017: Building Resilience for Peace and Food Security* (Rome, Italy: FAO, 2017), 35, www.fao.org/3/a-I7695e.pdf.

[4]World Food Program USA, *Winning the Peace: Hunger and Instability* (Washington, DC: WFPUSA, 2017), 7, www.wfpusa.org/winningthepeace.

[5]World Food Program USA, *Winning the Peace*, 8.

[6]"At the Root of Exodus: Food Security, Conflict and International Migration," World Food Progamme, May 2017, https://docs.wfp.org/api/documents/WFP-0000015358/download/?_ga=2.83696790.1070572661.1546420321-237976106.1532958898.

[7]"Journey to Extremism in Africa: Drivers, Incentives and the Tipping Point for Recruitment," United Nations Development Programme, 2017, https://journey-to-extremism.undp.org/content/downloads/UNDP-JourneyToExtremism-report-2017-english.pdf, 6.

[8]World Food Program USA, *Winning the Peace*, 31.

[9]"Global Military Spending Remains high at $1.7 Trillion," Stockholm International Peace Research Institute, May 2, 2018, www.sipri.org/media/press-release/2018/global-military-spending-remains-high-17-trillion.

[10]Alex Lockie, "Mattis Once Said If State Department Funding Gets Cut 'Then I Need to Buy More Ammunition,'" Business Insider, February 17, 2017, www.businessinsider.com/mattis-state-department-funding-need-to-buy-more-ammunition-2017-2?.

9. WHAT TO DO ABOUT MALNOURISHED PEOPLE AROUND THE WORLD (TONY CAMPOLO)

[1]Mark Doyle, "US Urged to Stop Haiti Rice Subsidies," BBC News, October 5, 2010, www.bbc.com/news/world-latin-america-11472874.

10. "REMEMBER US WHEN YOU COME INTO YOUR KINGDOM" (JEREMY K. EVERETT)

[1]Jeremy Everett, "On a Day of Plenty, Let These Words Resonate: Remember Us, When You Come into Your Kingdom," Dallas News, November 22, 2018, www.dallasnews.com/opinion/commentary/2018/11/22/day-plenty-let-words-resonateremember-us-come-kingdom.

[2]Alisha Coleman-Jensen, Matthew P. Rabbitt, Christian A. Gregory, and Anita Singh, "Household Food Security in the United States in 2016," United States Department of Agriculture, Economic Research Report 237,

September 2017, www.ers.usda.gov/webdocs/publications/84973/err-237
.pdf?v=42979.

[3] Alisha Coleman-Jensen and Mark Nord, "Food Insecurity Among Households with Working-Age Adults with Disabilities," United States Department of Agriculture, Economic Research Report 144, January 2013,
www.ers.usda.gov/webdocs/publications/45038/34589_err_144.pdf
?v=41284.

[4] US Department of Health and Human Services, "Nutrition and Overweight," chapter 19 in *Healthy People 2010* (Washington, DC: US Government Printing Office, 2000), www.cdc.gov/nchs/data/hpdata2010
/hp2010_final_review_focus_area_19.pdf.

[5] Robynn Cox and Sally Wallace, "The Impact of Incarceration on Food
Insecurity Among Households with Children," *Andrew Young School of
Policy Studies Research Paper Series* No. 13-05 (2013).

[6] John Cook, "Risk and Protective Factors Associated with Prevalence of
VLFS in Children among Children of Foreign-Born Mothers," *University
of Kentucky Center for Poverty Research Discussion Series* 20 (2013).

[7] Jung Sun Lee, Craig Gundersen, John Cook, Barbara Laraia, Mary Ann
Johnson. "Food Insecurity and Health Across the Lifespan." *Advances in
Nutrition* 3 (2012):44-74.

[8] Craig Hadley, Deborah L. Crooks, "Coping and the Biosocial Consequences of Food Insecurity in the 21st Century," *American Journal of
Physical Anthropology* 55 (2012):72-94.

[9] Coleman-Jensen, Rabbitt, Gregory, and Singh, "Household Food Security
in the United States in 2016."

[10] Jessica L. Semega, Kayla R. Fontenot, and Melissa A. Kollar, "Income and
Poverty in the United States: 2016," United States Census Bureau, September 2017, www.census.gov/content/dam/Census/library/publications
/2017/demo/P60-259.pdf.

[11] Semega, Fontenot, and Kollar, "Income and Poverty in the United
States: 2016."

[12] Coleman-Jensen, Rabbitt, Gregory, and Singh, "Household Food Security
in the United States in 2016."

[13] "Map the Meal Gap: Food Insecurity in the United States," Feeding
America, accessed March 27, 2019, http://map.feedingamerica.org.

[14]"Food insecurity is measured by the U.S. Household Food Security Survey Module, which has been in widespread use for nearly 20 years. It asks questions about respondents' reports of uncertain, insufficient, or inadequate food access, availability, and use because of limited financial resources, and about the compromised eating patterns and consumption that might result. The USDA uses the responses to classify households into four categories: high food security, marginal food security, low food security, and very low food security. Households with high or marginal food security are called *food secure*, and households with low or very low food security are called *food insecure*. To define hunger for this report, we chose a precise and readily available measure called *very low food security*, which occurs when eating patterns are disrupted or food intake is reduced for at least one household member because the household lacked money and other resources for food. . . . Thus, when we use the word 'hunger' we mean households experiencing *very low food security*." National Commission on Hunger, "Freedom from Hunger: An Achievable Goal for the United States of America," 2015, www.aei.org/wp-content/uploads/2016/01/Hunger_Commission _Final_Report.pdf.

[15]Coleman-Jensen, Rabbitt, Gregory, and Singh, "Household Food Security in the United States in 2016."

[16]Coleman-Jensen, Rabbitt, Gregory, and Singh, "Household Food Security in the United States in 2016."

[17]Hilary Seligman, Ann Bolger, David Guzman, Andrea Lopez, and Kirsten Bibbins-Domingo, "Exhaustion of Food Budgets at Month's End and Hospital Admissions for Hypoglycemia." *Health Affairs* 33 (2014): 116-23.

[18]"Public High School Graduation Rates" National Center for Education Statistics, updated May 2018, http://nces.ed.gov/programs/coe/indicator _coi.asp.

[19]Katherine Alaimo, Christine M. Olson, and Edward A. Frongillo Jr., "Food Insufficiency and American School-Aged Children's Cognitive, Academic, and Psychosocial Development," *American Academy of Pediatrics* 108 (2001): 44-53.

[20]Coleman-Jensen, Rabbitt, Gregory, and Singh, "Household Food Security in the United States in 2016."

[21]US Bureau of Labor Statistics, "Highlights of Women's Earnings in 2016," August 2017, www.bls.gov/opub/reports/womens-earnings/2016/pdf /home.pdf.

[22]Alisha Coleman-Jensen, Matthew P. Rabbitt, Christian A. Gregory, and Anita Singh, "Household Food Security in the United States in 2016," ERR-237, September 2017, www.ers.usda.gov/webdocs/publications /84973/err-237.pdf?v=42979.

11. CAUGHT IN CONFLICT (KIMBERLY FLOWERS)

[1]"Hunger Continues to Intensify in Conflict Zones, UN Agencies Report to Security Council," UN News, January 29, 2018, https://news.un.org/en /story/2018/01/1001471.

[2]"The State of Food Security and Nutrition in the World," Food and Agriculture Organization of the United Nations, accessed March 22, 2019, www.fao.org/state-of-food-security-nutrition/en.

[3]"Yemen—Complex Emergency," United States Agency of International Development, December 4, 2018, www.usaid.gov/sites/default/files /documents/1866/yemen_ce_fs03_12-04-2018.pdf.

[4]"Conflict Pushes South Sudanese into Hunger—More Than 6 Million People Face Desperate Food Shortages," UNICEF, September 28, 2018, www.unicef.org/press-releases/conflict-pushes-south-sudanese -hunger-more-6-million-people-face-desperate-food.

[5]Norman Borlaug, "Nobel Lecture," December 11, 1970, www.nobelprize .org/prizes/peace/1970/borlaug/lecture.

[6]Emmy Simmons, "Recurring Storms: Food Insecurity, Political Instability, and Conflict," Center for Strategic and International Studies, February 2017, https://csis-prod.s3.amazonaws.com/s3fs-public/publication /170124_Simmons_RecurringStorms_Web.pdf.

[7]Josh Rogin, "Rubio Makes the Case for Foreign Aid," Foreign Policy, July 5, 2011, https://foreignpolicy.com/2011/07/05/rubio-makes-the-case-for -foreign-aid.

[8]"Feed the Future," United States Agency of International Development, accessed March 22, 2019, www.usaid.gov/what-we-do/agriculture-and -food-security/increasing-food-security-through-feed-future.

[9]World Bank, *Piecing Together the Poverty Puzzle: Poverty and Shared Prosperity 2018* (Washington, DC: World Bank, 2018), https://openknowledge .worldbank.org/bitstream/handle/10986/30418/9781464813306.pdf, 38.

12. THE POSSIBLE IMPOSSIBLE DREAM
(GABE SALGUERO)

[1]Chris E. W. Green, *Surprised by God: How and Why What We Think about the Divine Matters* (Eugene, OR: Cascade Books, 2018), 60.

15. A THOUSAND DAYS AND A MILLION
QUESTIONS (CATHLEEN FALSANI)

[1]"Nutrition in the First 1,000 Days," Save the Children, May 2012, www .savethechildren.org/content/dam/usa/reports/advocacy/sowm/sowm -2012.pdf.

[2]"Infant Mortality Rate: Malawi," The United Nations Inter-agency Group for Child Mortality Estimation, https://childmortality.org/data, accessed May 2019.

[3]"The Cost of Hunger in Africa: The Social and Economic Impact of Child Undernutrition in Malawi," World Food Programme, May 13, 2015, https:// documents.wfp.org/stellent/groups/public/documents/newsroom /wfp274603.pdf.

[4]"The Cost of Hunger in Africa: The Social and Economic Impact of Child Undernutrition in Malawi."

19. FROM HUNGER TO HOLISTIC HEALTH
(ELIZABETH URIYO AND CHRISTOPHER DELVAILLE)

[1]"Weight-for-Age Percentiles: Boys, Birth to 36 Months" CDC, May 30, 2000, www.cdc.gov/growthcharts/data/set1/chart01.pdf.

[2]"Concepts and Definitions," chapter 3 in *Food Insecurity and Hunger in the United States: An Assessment of the Measure* (Washington, DC: The National Academies Press, 2006), www.nap.edu/read/11578/chapter/5.

[3]"Children: Reducing Mortality," World Health Organization, September 19, 2018, www.who.int/en/news-room/fact-sheets/detail/children-reducing -mortality.

[4]Food and Agriculture Organization of the United Nations, *The State of Food Security and Nutrition in the World 2017: Building Resilience for Peace and Food Security* (Rome, Italy: FAO, 2017), www.fao.org/3/a-I7787e.pdf.

[5]"High-Level Political Forum on Sustainable Development," United Nations, accessed May 2, 2019, https://sustainabledevelopment.un.org/hlpf /2017.

[6]"High-Level Political Forum on Sustainable Development."

[7]"High-Level Political Forum on Sustainable Development."

[8]"Speakers Urge Focus on Root Causes of Conflict as General Assembly Debates Strategies for Linking Sustainable Development, Lasting Peace," United Nations, January 24, 2017, www.un.org/press/en/2017/ga11884.doc .htm.

[9]"Speakers Urge Focus on Root Causes of Conflict."

23. FROM THE GARDEN TO THE TABLE (AMY GRANT)

[1]"Goal 2: Zero Hunger," United Nations Sustainable Development Goals, accessed April 2, 2019, www.un.org/sustainabledevelopment/hunger.

[2]"Global WASH Fast Facts," Centers for Disease Control and Prevention, accessed April 2, 2019, www.cdc.gov/healthywater/global/wash_statistics .html.

24. HUNGER, FASTING, AND FAITH
(ÁNGEL F. MÉNDEZ MONTOYA)

[1]"World Hunger Again on the Rise, Driven by Conflict and Climate Change, New UN Report Says," Food and Agriculture Organization of the United Nations, September 15, 2017, www.fao.org/news/story/en/item/1037253 /icode.

25. FEEDING THE HUNGRY BY RAISING DIGNITY
(KIMBERLY WILLIAMS-PAISLEY AND BRAD PAISLEY)

[1]Mark Twain, *The Complete Works of Mark Twain* (aka *Mark Twain's Notebook*) (New York: Harper & Bros, 1909), 328.

28. ENDING HUNGER STARTS WITH MODERNIZING
HOW WE DELIVER FOOD AID (BOB CORKER)

[1]Christopher B. Barrett, "Testimony before the United States Senate Committee on Foreign Relations Hearing on 'Modernizing the Food for Peace Program,'" Cornell University, October 19, 2017, www.foreign.senate .gov/imo/media/doc/101917_Barrett_Testimony.pdf.

[2]GAO, "International Food Assistance," June 2011, www.gao.gov/assets /330/320013.pdf.

29. EXODUS FROM HUNGER (DAVID BECKMANN)

[1]Committee on Labor and Public Welfare, US Senate, *Poverty, Hunger, and Federal Programs Background Information* (Washington, DC: US GPO, 1967).

[2]Arloc Sherman, Sharon Parrott, and Danlio Trisi, "Chart Book: The War on Poverty at 50," Center on Budget and Policy Priorities, January 7, 2014, www.cbpp.org/research/chart-book-the-war-on-poverty-at-50-overview.

[3]Feed the Future, "A Decade of Progress: Feed the Future Snapshot," accessed April 9, 2019, www.usaid.gov/sites/default/files/documents/1867/2018-ftf-snaphot.pdf, 5.

[4]"Stunting prevalence 1990-2017," UNICEF, WHO, World Bank Group Joint Malnutrition Estimates, May 2018 Edition, data.worldbank.org.

[5]Robert D. Putnam and David E. Campbell, *American Grace* (New York: Simon & Schuster, 2010).

GLOSSARY

[1]"Definitions of Food Insecurity," USDA, accessed May 2, 2019, www.ers.usda.gov/topics/food-nutrition-assistance/food-security-in-the-us/definitions-of-food-security.

CONTRIBUTORS

CHEF RICK BAYLESS

Most people know Rick Bayless from winning the title of Bravo's *Top Chef Masters* with his authentic Mexican cuisine. His highly rated public television series, *Mexico–One Plate at a Time*, has earned him multiple Daytime Emmy nominations for Best Culinary Host.

Chef Bayless is the author of nine cookbooks. His second, *Mexican Kitchen,* won the Julia Child IACP cookbook of the year award in 1996, and his fourth, *Mexico–One Plate at a Time*, won the James Beard Best International Cookbook of the Year award in 2001.

Chef Bayless established the Frontera Farmer Foundation in 2003 to support small Midwestern farms. To date, the Foundation has awarded nearly two hundred grants totaling nearly $2 million. In 2007 Rick was named the Humanitarian of the Year by the International Association of Culinary Professionals for his many philanthropic endeavors.

Chef Bayless has received a great number of James Beard Award nominations in many categories, and he has won seven, including Midwest Chef of the Year, National Chef of the Year, and Humanitarian of the Year. The government of Mexico has bestowed on Rick the Mexican Order of the Aztec Eagle–the highest decoration bestowed on foreigners whose work has benefitted Mexico and its people.

DAVID BEASLEY

In a public service and business career that spans more than four decades, David Beasley, executive director of the World Food Programme, has worked across political, religious, and ethnic lines to champion economic development, humanitarian assistance, education, and intercultural and interfaith cooperation for the most vulnerable people across the globe.

For the past decade, Mr. Beasley has worked with influential leaders and on-the-ground program managers in more than one hundred countries on projects to foster peace, reconciliation, and economic progress. Mr. Beasley also has helped strengthen cooperation and communication among the business, political, and nongovernmental sectors in regions of long-standing political, ethnic, and religious tension.

Mr. Beasley, who served as governor of South Carolina from 1995 to 1999, earned his bachelor's degree from Clemson University and a Doctor of Jurisprudence degree from the University of South Carolina, and also taught at the Harvard University Kennedy School of Government. He was elected first to public office at the age of twenty-one as a member of the South Carolina House of Representatives. He is married to the former Mary Wood Payne and is the father of four children.

DAVID BECKMANN

World Food Prize laureate David Beckmann is one of the foremost US advocates for ending hunger. As president of Bread for the World, he leads large-scale campaigns to strengthen US political commitment to overcome hunger in the United States and around the world. Bread for the World is a US Christian advocacy movement.

Mr. Beckmann is also president of Bread for the World Institute, which provides policy analysis on hunger and strategies to end it. He is founder and president of the Alliance to End Hunger, which engages diverse US institutions—Muslim and Jewish groups, corporations, unions, and universities—in building the political will to end hunger.

Mr. Beckmann has served on the President's Advisory Council on Faith-Based and Neighborhood Partnerships, USAID's Advisory Committee on Voluntary Foreign Aid, the US Trade Representative's Advisory Committee on Africa, the Executive Committee of the Modernizing Foreign Assistance Network, and the Council on Foreign Relations.

Mr. Beckmann is a Lutheran pastor and an economist. Prior to joining Bread, he worked at the World Bank for fifteen years, overseeing development projects and driving innovations to make the Bank more effective in reducing poverty.

DIANE BLACK

As a registered nurse, small-businesswoman, and former educator, Representative Diane Black (R-TN) brought a unique perspective to her work in Congress. Her faith in America's promise was shaped from an early age. The daughter of Great Depression–era parents, Ms. Black spent the earliest years of her life in public housing and would go on to become the first person in her family to earn a college education.

In Congress, Ms. Black served as chairman of the House Budget Committee, where she led the passage of the 2018 fiscal year budget that cut billions of dollars in wasteful spending and confronted the crippling debt burden in Washington. Diane also served on the House Ways and Means Committee and quickly established herself as a leader in the efforts to reform the US tax code for the first time in over three decades.

Through her more than forty years of experience working in the health care field, Ms. Black learned first-hand about the importance of high-quality care and the obstacles faced by patients, health care providers, and employers. Her real world experiences as a nurse uniquely positioned her as a credible and effective leader on health care policy in Congress. Although a nurse, Diane was a welcomed member of the

Doctor's Caucus engaging in health care discussions with physician Congressional colleagues.

TONY CAMPOLO

Tony Campolo is professor emeritus of sociology at Eastern University and a former faculty member at the University of Pennsylvania. For forty years, he led the Evangelical Association for the Promotion of Education, an organization which he founded to create and support programs serving needy communities.

More recently, Dr. Campolo has provided leadership for the progressive Christian movement Red Letter Christians as well as for the Campolo Center for Ministry, a program which provides support to those the church has called to full-time ministry.

In November 2012, Dr. Campolo received a Lifetime Achievement Award from the National Youth Worker's Convention. The wording on the award said, "Award of Lifetime Achievement is proudly presented to Tony Campolo who has defined and courageously pioneered what it means to encourage, care, and lead students, possessing the qualities that inspire us and provoke us to continue the journey into the future with boldness and confidence. As a result of Tony's life of ministry and leadership he has left a legacy of encouragement and hope to youth workers and students everywhere."

BOB CORKER

Bob Corker is a successful businessman and former United States Senator. He was previously named one of the 100 most influential people in the world by *TIME* magazine. Corker represented Tennesseans in the Senate from 2007 to 2018, where he served as chairman of the Senate Foreign Relations Committee and was an active member of the Senate Banking Committee and Senate Budget Committee. He was Tennessee's commissioner of finance and mayor of Chattanooga before being elected to the Senate, but he spent most of his life in business. That results-driven businessman's perspective allowed him to make a mark early in his Senate tenure and become a pragmatic thought leader on fiscal, financial, and foreign relations issues.

As an advocate for using limited foreign aid dollars more efficiently to advance US interests, Senator Corker has led efforts to modernize emergency food assistance programs in a way that will eliminate waste and inefficiencies to help more people in need.

CHRISTOPHER DELVAILLE

Christopher Delvaille has served at Compassion International for more than thirteen years. Currently, he is the Senior Strategy and Planning Advisor for the Global Program Group, developing strategy management frameworks and tools for the function responsible for program design and implementation.

Earlier in his career at Compassion, Mr. Delvaille served as director of Compassion's Office of Corporate Planning, where he led an annual planning process and managed the ministry's balanced scorecard and strategy management process.

Prior to his time at Compassion, he was the Manager of Policy and Planning for the Providence Housing Authority in Rhode Island, where he provided oversight of the agency's five-year strategic planning process, annual planning, goals management planning, and program and project analysis.

Mr. Delvaille holds a master's degree in community planning from the University of Rhode Island, and a bachelor's degree in government from Connecticut College.

JENNY EATON DYER

Jenny Eaton Dyer, PhD, is the founder of The 2030 Collaborative. Formerly, she worked with Senator William H. Frist, MD, as the executive director of Hope Through Healing Hands. She continues to direct the Faith-Based Coalition for Global Nutrition with support from the Eleanor Crook Foundation. Dyer is a lecturer in the Department of Health Policy at Vanderbilt University Medical Center teaching global health politics and policy. She also is a lecturer at Vanderbilt School of Divinity teaching religion and global health.

Ms. Dyer formerly served as the National Faith Outreach Director for the DATA Foundation and the ONE Campaign, Bono's organization, from 2003 to 2008.

Ms. Dyer has written many academic articles and opinion pieces on the intersection of religion and health. She is a contributor to the book *Why Save Africa: Answers from Around the World* (Hatherleigh Press, 2011) and a cocompiler of *The Mother & Child Project: Raising Our Voices for Health and Hope* (Zondervan, 2015) and *The aWAKE Project: Uniting Against the African AIDS Crisis* (W Pub Group, 2002).

JEREMY K. EVERETT

Jeremy K. Everett is the founder and executive director of the Texas Hunger Initiative (THI), a capacity-building, anti-hunger project within Baylor University. THI partners with the US Department of Agriculture, Texas state agencies, and numerous faith- and community-based organizations to develop and implement strategies to alleviate hunger through research, policy analysis, education, and community organizing.

Prior to THI, Mr. Everett worked for international and community development organizations as a teacher, religious leader, community organizer, and organic farmer. He frequently delivers presentations to churches, nonprofit organizations, universities, and the government sector about hunger and poverty.

Mr. Everett earned a bachelor's degree from Samford University and a Master of Divinity from Baylor University. Jeremy is a Next

Generation Fellow of the University of Texas LBJ School's Strauss Center for International Security and Law and a Senior Fellow with World Hunger Relief, Inc., and was recently appointed by US Congress to serve on the National Commission on Hunger.

Mr. Everett is married to Amy Miley Everett. They have three sons: Lucas, Sam, and Wyatt.

CATHLEEN FALSANI

Cathleen Falsani is a longtime religion journalist and author, specializing in the intersection of faith and culture. From 2000 to 2010, Ms. Falsani was the religion writer and columnist for the *Chicago Sun-Times*, and is the Faith & Values Columnist for the *Orange County Register*. She is a longtime correspondent for Religion News Service and a featured writer for Sojourners, where she was the director of new media from 2010 to 2012.

In addition to her work covering religion in the United States and abroad, Ms. Falsani has written extensively about global poverty, AIDS and HIV in sub-Saharan Africa, and other issues affecting the developing world.

In 2005, Ms. Falsani received the James O. Supple Religion Writer of the Year award from the Religion Newswriters Association, and she twice has been a finalist for the Templeton Religion Reporter of the Year award. She serves as a member of the Advisory Board for Girls and Women at the ONE Campaign. She lives in Southern California with her husband, the journalist and author Maurice Possley, and their college-aged son, Vasco Fitzmaurice Mark David Possley.

WILLIAM H. FRIST

William H. Frist is a heart and lung transplant surgeon and former US Senate Majority Leader. He is a partner at health services investment firm Cressey & Company and founding partner at Frist Cressey

Ventures, where he works to solve health care's most pressing challenges with innovative private sector solutions.

Senator Frist represented Tennessee in the US Senate for twelve years and was elected Majority Leader in 2003. His leadership was instrumental in the passage of the 2003 Medicare Modernization Act and the historic PEPFAR HIV/AIDS legislation that has saved millions of lives worldwide.

Dedicated to furthering health and healing through service, he founded Hope Through Healing Hands, a humanitarian organization devoted to improving global health; NashvilleHealth, a community collaborative focused on improving the health of Nashvillians; and Tennessee's State Collaborative on Reforming Education (SCORE).

He serves on the boards of publicly-traded companies AECOM, Select Medical Corporation, and Teladoc, as well as on the boards of the Robert Wood Johnson Foundation, The Nature Conservancy, Kaiser Family Foundation, and others.

KIMBERLY FLOWERS

Kimberly Flowers is director of the CSIS Global Food Security Project, which examines and highlights the impact of food security on US strategic global interests. The project evaluates current efforts and provides long-term, strategic guidance to policymakers to ensure that US foreign assistance programs are efficient, effective, and sustainable.

Prior to joining CSIS in 2015, Ms. Flowers was the communications director for Fintrac, an international development company focusing on hunger eradication and poverty alleviation through agricultural solutions. From 2005 to 2011, she worked for the US Agency for International Development, serving overseas as a development, outreach, and communications officer in Ethiopia and Jamaica, supporting public affairs in Haiti directly after the 2010 earthquake, and leading strategic communications for the US government's global hunger and nutrition initiative, Feed the Future.

Ms. Flowers began her international development career in 1999 as a Peace Corps volunteer in Bulgaria, where she founded a young women's leadership camp that continues today. She is a magna cum laude graduate of William Jewell College, studied at Oxford University, and is an alumna of the Pryor Center for Leadership Development.

HELENE GAYLE

Helene Gayle is president and CEO of The Chicago Community Trust, one of the nation's leading community foundations. The Trust works with donors, nonprofits, community leaders, and residents to lead and inspire philanthropic efforts that improve the quality of life in the Chicago region.

Previously, Dr. Gayle was CEO of McKinsey Social Initiative, a non-profit that builds partnerships for social impact. For almost a decade, she was president and CEO of CARE, a leading international humanitarian organization. An expert on global development, humanitarian and health issues, Dr. Gayle spent twenty years with the Centers for Disease Control, working primarily on HIV/AIDS. She also worked at the Bill & Melinda Gates Foundation, directing programs on HIV/AIDS and other global health issues.

Named one of *Forbes's* "100 Most Powerful Women," she has authored numerous articles on global and domestic public health issues, poverty alleviation, gender equality, and social justice.

Dr. Gayle was born and raised in Buffalo, NY. She earned a BA in psychology at Barnard College, an MD at the University of Pennsylvania, and an MPH at Johns Hopkins University. She has received fifteen honorary degrees and holds faculty appointments at the University of Washington and Emory University.

AMY GRANT

Conventional wisdom has it that Amy Grant put Contemporary Christian Music on the map, becoming the first CCM artist to have a platinum record, the first to hit No. 1 on the pop charts, and the first to perform at the Grammy Awards. Since then, Grant has been strumming her way through a thirty-plus-year adventure as a singer-songwriter, author, television host, and speaker.

Grant has sold more than thirty million albums worldwide, including three multi-platinum, six platinum, and four gold. Her chart performance has also been consistent throughout her career, boasting six No. 1 hits, 10 "Top 40" pop singles, 17 "Top 40" adult contemporary tracks, and multiple contemporary Christian chart-toppers. In recognition of such success, Ms. Grant has received six Grammy awards and twenty-six Dove awards, a star on the Hollywood Walk of Fame, a star on the Music City Walk of Fame, and induction into the Gospel Music Hall of Fame in Nashville.

Ms. Grant resides with her family in Nashville, Tennessee, and is widely known for her philanthropy and tireless involvement in local causes and charitable organizations. Her own organization, The Helping Hands Foundation, has afforded her the opportunity to identify needs around her and the resources to help meet them.

TONY P. HALL

Three times nominated for the Nobel Peace Prize, Ambassador Tony P. Hall is a leading advocate for hunger relief programs and improving human rights conditions in the world.

Hall served as the United States Ambassador to the United Nations Agencies for Food and Agriculture. He retired from official diplomatic service in April 2006, and currently serves as the executive director of the Alliance to End Hunger, which engages diverse institutions in building the public and political will to end hunger at home and abroad.

Prior to his diplomatic service, Ambassador Hall represented the Third District of Ohio in the US Congress for almost twenty-four years. During his tenure, he was chairman of the House Select Committee on Hunger and the Democratic Caucus Task Force on Hunger. He founded the Congressional Friends of Human Rights Monitors and authored legislation that supported food aid, child survival, basic education, primary health care, microenterprise, and development assistance in the world's poorest countries. Ambassador Hall also founded and chaired the Congressional Hunger Center, a non-governmental organization committed to ending hunger through training and educational programs for emerging leaders. A founding member of the Select Committee on Hunger, Ambassador Hall served as its chairman from 1989 to 1993.

RUDO KWARAMBA-KAYOMBO

Rudo Kwaramba-Kayombo is the Africa executive director for the ONE Campaign. Prior to joining ONE, she was country director for World Vision in Zimbabwe and Uganda, director of advocacy, communications, and education with World Vision UK, and regional director for Southern Africa for World Vision International, where she oversaw nine countries and ran diverse development, advocacy, and emergency response programs across the region.

She is a human rights lawyer by profession and holds a master of arts in public policy and administration from the University of York.

In 2005, Ms. Kwaramba-Kayombo was one of several spokes-persons for the Make Poverty History coalition campaign. She has served as an executive board member for Women in Law and Development in Africa and as a trustee of the Gateway Trust, a trust managing a Christian education group of schools in Harare. She has also been a member of the advisory board for the United Nations Development Programme for the Government of Zimbabwe's Capacity Building Project on Conflict Transformation.

NIKOLE LIM

Nikole Lim is a speaker and educator on leveraging dignity through the restorative art of storytelling.

From documenting a widow with leprosy in the jungles of Vietnam to providing scholarships for survivors of sexual violence in Zambia, furthering social justice through the arts has been a vital part of Ms. Lim's vocational journey. By using film and photography, she shifts paradigms on how stories are told by platforming voices of the oppressed—sharing stories of immense beauty arising out of seemingly broken situations.

Ms. Lim is the cofounder and international director of Freely in Hope, a nonprofit organization that equips survivors and advocates to lead in ending the cycle of sexual violence. Freely in Hope operates in Kenya and Zambia, providing psychological counseling, health care, and high school and university scholarships for young women.

Ms. Lim is part of the Red Letter Christians network. She consults regularly with international organizations including the Salvation Army, has spoken in faith-based initiatives at the United Nations Women Conference, and lectures at universities across the United States.

JONATHAN MARTIN

While the product of the sweat and sawdust of the tent revival, Rev. Jonathan Martin believes in a big, wide tent, where all of you is welcome, and he preaches a love that is hotter than fire and brimstone. At six-feet-five-inches tall, he is known for his commanding frame and bold preaching, but also a voice made tender from his own experience of finding God on the underside.

Presently the pastor of a new congregation, The Table in Oklahoma City, Rev. Martin is the author of two acclaimed books, *Prototype* and *How to Survive a Shipwreck*. He has served as a pastor, church planter, and an activist. Wherever he goes, the message is always the same: no matter who you are, where you've been, or what you've done—God is at work to bring beauty out of your brokenness. He has carried this message to churches, universities and seminaries, and conferences and retreats all over the globe.

The Reverend Martin's work and/or words have been featured in media such as the *New York Times*, the *Atlantic*, NPR, *Newsweek*, Vox, *Sojourners*, the *Huffington Post*, and *Relevant* magazine, and he has published in scholarly journals including the *Journal of Pentecostal Theology*.

MIKE McHARGUE

Mike McHargue (better known as "Science Mike") is an author, podcaster, and speaker who travels the world helping people understand the science of life's most profound and mundane experiences.

His bestselling debut book, *Finding God in the Waves*, has helped thousands of readers understand faith in the twenty-first century. Mr. McHargue is the host of the Ask Science Mike podcast, and cofounded The Liturgists Podcast with his friend Michael Gungor. He recently has appeared before sold-out audiences in New York, Chicago, and London, and has bylines in *Relevant* magazine, Storyline, BioLogos, and the *Washington Post*.

ÁNGEL F. MÉNDEZ MONTOYA

Ángel F. Méndez Montoya is a scholar, Dominican friar (Order of Preachers) of the US Southern Dominican Province, and author of *The Theology of Food: Eating and the Eucharist* (Wiley-Blackwell, 2012). He is a professor in the department of religious sciences of the Universidad Iberoamericana in Mexico City and was coordinator of the Fe y Culture there. He teaches courses, seminars, and conferences in various universities and academic institutes in Mexico and abroad.

Dr. Méndez Montoya's writing has appeared in several scholarly anthologies and in national and international journals, including *Christus* magazine, *Annals of Anthropology*, *New Black-Friars*, *Concillium*, *CrossCurrents*, *Wort Und Antwort*, *Modern Theology*, and *The Bible in Transmission*.

Born in Mexicali, Mexico, Méndez Montoya earned his PhD in philosophical theology from the University of Virginia and wrote his doctoral thesis as a scholar in residence at the University of Cambridge in the United Kingdom. His dissertation, "The Theology of Food: Eating and the Eucharist," was nominated for the Michael Ramsey Prize in 2011 and published in Spanish under the title "Festín del deseo: hacia una teología alimentaria."

WILL MOORE

William Moore has served as executive director of The Eleanor Crook Foundation since 2015.

He was formerly chief storyteller at the United Nations Millennium Campaign, where he helped coordinate UN country office engagement plans for the Sustainable Development Goals, and worked to highlight the human aspect of data and development.

Mr. Moore serves on the board of directors for Bread for the World and the Alliance to End Hunger, as well as the advisory board for the Centre for Innovation and Health at Concern Worldwide. A North Carolina native, Mr. Moore graduated with top marks from Columbia University with a degree in American Studies.

BRAD PAISLEY

Brad Paisley is a critically acclaimed singer, songwriter, guitarist, and entertainer whose talents have earned him numerous awards, including three Grammys, two American Music Awards, fourteen Academy of Country Music Awards, and fourteen Country Music

Association Awards (including Entertainer of the Year), among many others. He has been a proud member of the Grand Ole Opry since 2001.

A native of West Virginia, Mr. Paisley released his first album, *Who Needs Pictures*, in 1999. The album went platinum and catapulted him to fame. In 2001, Mr. Paisley met the actress Kimberly Williams after writing a song with lyrics about meeting her. He made a video to accompany the single, and Williams agreed to appear.

The couple married in 2003, and welcomed their first child, William "Huck" Huckleberry in 2007, and their second child, Jasper Warren, in 2009. He resides with his family in Tennessee.

SAMUEL RODRIGUEZ

Rev. Dr. Samuel Rodriguez is president of the National Hispanic Christian Leadership Conference (NHCLC), the world's largest Hispanic Christian organization with 40,118 US churches and more than 450,000 churches spread throughout the Spanish-speaking diaspora.

Pastor Rodriguez has been named among the "Top 100 Christian Leaders in America" by *Newsmax* in 2018, and *TIME* nominated him as one of the "100 most influential people in the world" in 2013. He is regularly featured in the *Washington Post, CNN, Fox News, Univision, ABC, PBS, Christianity Today, Newsweek*, the *New York Times*, the *Wall Street Journal*, and other media outlets.

Pastor Rodriguez has advised Presidents Bush, Obama, and Trump, and frequently consults with members of both political parties in Congress to advance immigration and criminal justice reforms as well as religious freedom initiatives. In January 2017, Rodriguez became the first Latino Evangelical to participate in a presidential swearing-in ceremony.

Pastor Rodriguez serves as cofounder and lead pastor of TBN Salsa, an international Christian-based broadcast television network. He also serves as senior pastor of New Season Christian Worship Center in Sacramento, California.

JEFFREY D. SACHS

Jeffrey D. Sachs is a world-renowned professor of economics, leader in sustainable development, senior United Nations adviser, bestselling author, and syndicated columnist whose monthly newspaper columns appear in more than one hundred countries. The *New York Times* has dubbed him "probably the most important economist in the world." A recent survey by the *Economist* ranked him as among the world's three most influential living economists of the past decade.

Professor Sachs serves as the director of the Center for Sustainable Development at Columbia University. He is University Professor at Columbia University, the university's highest academic rank.

Professor Sachs is special adviser to United Nations Secretary-General António Guterres on the Sustainable Development Goals, and previously advised UN Secretary-General Ban Ki-moon on both the Sustainable Development Goals and Millennium Development Goals and UN Secretary-General Kofi Annan on the Millennium Development Goals. He is a Distinguished Fellow of the International Institute of Applied Systems Analysis in Laxenburg, Austria.

He is currently director of the UN Sustainable Development Solutions Network, and a Commissioner of the ITU/UNESCO Broadband Commission for Development. Professor Sachs is Chair and Founder of SDG USA, a non-governmental initiative to promote the Sustainable Development Goal concepts in the United States.

GABE SALGUERO

Rev. Dr. Gabe Salguero is the founder and president of the National Latino Evangelical Coalition (NALEC). He and his wife, Rev. Jeanette Salguero, are pastors at Calvario City Church in Orlando, Florida.

Pastor Salguero is a sought-after evangelical leader and has been featured in media coverage by CNN, the *Washington Post*, the *New York Times*, and *TIME* magazine. He is the former Director of the Institute of Faith and Public Life at Princeton Theological Seminary.

Pastor Salguero has been recognized for his work on behalf of poor and vulnerable communities in the United States and abroad. He formerly served on the White House Faith-Based Advisory Council on issues including immigration, poverty, and refugees.

MARK K. SHRIVER

Mark K. Shriver is the senior vice president of US Programs and Advocacy at Save the Children, an organization that reaches America's most vulnerable children through early education, literacy, health care, and disaster preparedness. He also serves as chief executive officer of Save the Children Action Network, where he leads an effort to mobilize Americans to end preventable maternal, newborn, and child deaths globally, and to ensure that every child in the United States has access to high-quality early childhood education.

Mr. Shriver has made his career fighting for social justice in advocacy and service organizations, as well as elected office, and has focused on advancing the right of every child to a safe and vibrant childhood. He was a member of the Maryland House of Delegates from 1994 to 2002. He joined Save the Children in 2003, serving as senior vice president for US Programs until 2013 and then resuming that role again in 2017.

RON SIDER

Ronald Sider is Senior Distinguished Professor of Theology, Holistic Ministry, and Public Policy at Palmer Theological Seminary and president emeritus of Evangelicals for Social Action.

A widely known evangelical speaker and writer, Mr. Sider has spoken on six continents and published more than thirty books and scores of articles. In 1982, the *Christian Century* named him one of the twelve "most influential persons in the field of religion in the US." His *Rich Christians in an Age of Hunger* (Thomas Nelson, reprint 2015) was recognized by *Christianity Today* as one of the one hundred most influential religious books of the twentieth century and named the seventh most influential book in the evangelical world in the past fifty years. He was the publisher of *PRISM* magazine and a contributing editor of *Christianity Today* for twenty years, and is a contributing editor for *Sojourners*.

Mr. Sider holds a PhD from Yale University, and has lectured at scores of colleges and universities around the world, including Yale, Harvard, Princeton, and Oxford. In 2014, he received the William Sloane Coffin Award for Peace and Justice from Yale Divinity School.

RACHEL MARIE STONE

Rachel Marie Stone is the author of several books, including *Eat With Joy: Redeeming God's Gift of Food* (InterVarsity Press, 2013), which won the *Christianity Today* book award in the category of Christian Living, and was named one of Religion News Service's "Top Ten Intriguing Books of 2013."

Ms. Stone also did extensive revisions to the classic *More-With-Less: A World Cookbook*, the Mennonite cookbook that weds faith, justice, simplicity, and good eating—all the things she cares about very much. The revised edition was published in 2016 by Herald Press.

Ms. Stone is a regular contributor to *Christianity Today's* women's blog, *Her.meneutics*, and serves on the editorial board for *Christianity Today*. Her writing has appeared in a host of publications. She contributed an essay to the book *Talking Taboo: American Christian Women Get Frank About Faith* (White Cloud Press, 2013), and a chapter to the book

Disquiet Time: Rants and Reflections on the Good Book by the Skeptical, the Faithful, and a Few Scoundrels (Hachette, 2014), coedited by Cathleen Falsani.

Ms. Stone lives in the northeastern United States with her husband of more than thirteen years, Tim, with whom she has two Lego-obsessed boys.

ROGER THUROW

Roger Thurow joined the Chicago Council on Global Affairs as senior fellow for global food and agriculture in 2010 after three decades at the *Wall Street Journal*.

For twenty years, he served as a *Journal* foreign correspondent, based in Europe and Africa. His coverage of global affairs spanned the Cold War, the reunification of Germany, the release of Nelson Mandela, the end of apartheid, the wars in the former Yugoslavia, and the humanitarian crises of the first decade of this century—along with ten Olympic Games.

In 2003, he and *Journal* colleague Scott Kilman wrote a series of stories on famine in Africa that was a finalist for the Pulitzer Prize in International Reporting. Mr. Thurow and Mr. Kilman are authors of the book, *Enough: Why the World's Poorest Starve in an Age of Plenty*. In 2009, they were awarded Action Against Hunger's Humanitarian Award.

In May 2012, Mr. Thurow published his second book, *The Last Hunger Season: A Year in an African Farm Community on the Brink of Change*.

His latest book, *The First 1,000 Days: A Crucial Time for Mothers and Children—And the World*, chronicles the importance of good nutrition for maternal and infant health.

STEVE TAYLOR

Steve Taylor is a filmmaker and recording artist. His latest movie, *Blue Like Jazz*, premiered at the South By Southwest Film Festival, was released theatrically by Roadside Attractions, and won the 2013 Wilbur Award for Best Feature Film, joining past winners *Hidden Figures, The Help, Schindler's List,* and *Dead Man Walking.*

Mr. Taylor is a multiple Grammy Award nominee and one-fifth of the rock band Steve Taylor & the Danielson Foil, whose latest project— *Wow to the Deadness*—was recorded by famed punk rock producer Steve Albini.

He is the filmmaker-in-residence at Lipscomb University and lives in Nashville with his wife, the artist D. L. Taylor, and their daughter, Sarah. You can follow him on Twitter @theperfectfoil and *stevetaylorpresents.com.*

ELIZABETH URIYO

Elizabeth Uriyo serves as senior vice president of Compassion International's Global Leadership Office. In this role, Ms. Uriyo is responsible for facilitating Compassion's multi-year strategy and strategy execution, running presidential office operations, and leading global corporate communications. Prior to this role, she was senior director of Compassion's Global Program group (which serves 1.8 million children living in poverty in twenty-five countries in Africa, Asia, and Central and South America), where she provided day-to-day leadership of strategy, resource allocation, monitoring, administration, project completion, and information technology.

She holds a master's degree in business administration from the University of Chicago's Booth School of Business and a PhD and Master of Science degree in grain science and industry from Kansas State University.

A native of Tanzania, Ms. Uriyo spent much of her childhood in Nigeria. Growing up, she supported her mother's involvement with organizations caring for motherless and disabled children, which greatly influenced her desire to serve children in poverty.

KIMBERLY WILLIAMS-PAISLEY

Kimberly Williams-Paisley has been starring in film, television, and theater for more than twenty-five years. Now a *New York Times* bestselling author for her book *Where the Light Gets In*, which chronicles the impact of her mother Linda's dementia, Ms. Williams-Paisley has garnered praise and admiration across the film, television, and publishing arenas.

Ms. Williams-Paisley first lit up the screen as the radiant young bride in the comedy feature film series *Father of the Bride* and *Father of the Bride Part II*. She went on to star in such films as *How to Eat Fried Worms*, *We Are Marshall*, and *Undiscovered Gyrl*. Ms. Williams-Paisley has starred many television shows. She made her Broadway debut in the Tony Award-winning *The Last Night of Ballyhoo*.

Ms. Williams-Paisley is a spokesperson for the Alzheimer's Association, is actively involved with JP/HRO, Sean Penn's Haitian relief organization, which currently is working to improve the lives of the people of Port-au-Prince. She also is a member of the Entertainment Council for Feeding America, a Nashville Zoo Board member, and a supporter of various animal rescue organizations.

She has been married to Brad Paisley since 2003, and they have two young sons, Huck and Jasper. The family lives in Tennessee.